OXFORD MEDICAL PUBLICATIONS

Health Behaviour Research and Health Promotion

Health Behaviour Research and Health Promotion

Oxford University Press, Walton Street, Oxford OX2 6DP
Oxford New York Toronto
Delhi Bombay Calcutta Madras Karachi
Petaling Jaya Singapore Hong Kong Tokyo
Nairobi Dar es Salaam Cape Town
Melbourne Auckland
and associated companies in
Berlin Ibadan

Oxford is a trade mark of Oxford University Press

Published in the United States
by Oxford University Press, New York

British Library Cataloguing in Publication Data
Health behaviour research and
health promotion.
1. Man. Health. Self-care
I. Anderson, Robert, 1944–
613
ISBN 0-19-261600-5

Library of Congress Cataloging in Publication Data
Health behaviour research and health promotion.
Includes bibliographies and index.
1. Health behavior.   2. Health promotion.
I. Anderson, Robert, 1944–   .
RA776.9.R65   1988   613   88-15172
ISBN 0-19-261600-5

Set by Joshua Associates Ltd., Oxford
Printed in Great Britain by
Biddles Ltd, Guildford and King's Lynn

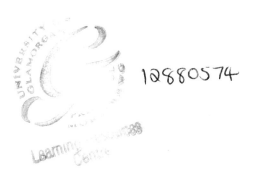

Foreword

Professor Raymond Illsley

Formerly Director of the Medical Research Council Medical Sociology Unit,
University of Aberdeen

Some disciplines and clinical specialities seem never to change in their essential meaning. There is a simple generic similarity between the barber-surgeons of the nineteenth century and today's sophisticated surgeons. Everybody knew and knows that they open you up, re-arrange your components and sew you up again. The skills, the technology, the range of operations and, above all, the survival rates have changed enormously but surgery is essentially the same. Other disciplines, such as public health, change their name frequently (epidemiology, preventive medicine, social medicine, community medicine) and sometimes change of name also implies change of function. This is outstandingly true of health promotion. Only a decade ago it was usually called health education, it has subsequently hesitated between disease prevention and even health prevention, and has finally (temporarily) settled down as health promotion. These changes have not occurred at random. They reflect fast and fundamental changes in content, understanding, and status.

After the epidemics and the public health successes of the late nineteenth century came the inter-war and post-war advances in pharmacology and the reduced threat of infection in the Western industrial world. The earlier consciousness that ill-health came from the physical and social environment and could be avoided by public health knowledge lost its strength and was replaced by implicit reliance upon individual treatment and the use of advanced techniques based upon the laboratory sciences. Epidemiology and public health became social medicine, and social hygiene was replaced by health education. The assumption was that individuals were unaware of the possibilities of treatment and care and, to a lesser extent, of behavioural risks. Education of the individual would create greater knowledge and awareness and would motivate people to seek treatment and to seek it at the right time. This simple theory took public health out of political action and, to a large extent, out of medicine for which it became a supportive and low status adjunct.

The contributions to this volume reveal an astonishing theoretical transformation which has occurred in little more than a decade. There is rightly much discussion about definitions and terminology, but more about theories, concepts, and policy. Education and individual action remain as important components of health promotion programmes and of health-related behaviour. They take their place, however, in a wider conception of causation and intervention. The individual is seen to be a part of a group, of a culture, of an eco-system, receiving signals and experiencing pressures which influence perceptions and valuation of health, and condition responses to health-related knowledge. Such groups, cultures, eco-systems and their associated values and behaviour, however, are seen, not as phenomena in their own right but as social creations, the outcome of history and geography, but more importantly of economic and social policies. Harmful exposure rarely occurs by accident; it is the result of the actions of others in pursuit of their own ends, whether these be governments, industries, private groups, or individuals: or the result of acts of omission, by the same wide range of agents, where awareness of harmful effects exists but counter-action, for many reasons, is avoided. Responsibility for today's equivalent of the open sewers of nineteenth-century Europe (still open in many areas of the world) is thus widespread. It must rest primarily with governments because they alone have comprehensive responsibility and powers, and because what they themselves create or permit by direct action, taxation, and regulation, through economic strategies or through health and social policies, must constitute in any society the greatest part of avoidable illness and death. Ultimate state responsibility does not confer moral immunity on all other organizations, groups, and individuals whose collective and individual behaviour creates risks for others.

The implications for research are both exciting and appalling. Research must extend across the sectors of governments (and blocks of governments); international and national trade and industry; organizations, professions, and groups concerned with health, social welfare, education, law, etc., to the social relationships of small groups and of individuals. It must deal with these not singly but in interaction; with causes of ill-health; with behaviour, culture, opinion, and attitude. It requires the involvement of an equally wide range of disciplines, not merely those of the health and social sciences, but the physical, industrial, and legal sciences. The principal victims of avoidable ill-health are largely poor and powerless individuals, groups, and countries: because they are partially responsible for their own behaviour they need to be studied and they are classically easy targets for researchers. The emphasis of research must, however, lie with the structures and institutions of our society, with the more powerful groups and organizations whose actions have effect on the health of millions and whose participation in health promotion is essential.

This volume moves towards an informed formulation of the issues, and towards a set of research priorities. It marks an important stage in the development of a fundamental programme of research and action.

Preface

This book is the result of a joint enterprise between the European Office of the World Health Organization and one of its Collaborating Centres—the Scottish Health Education Group. As part of SHEG's collaborative work-plan with WHO, a symposium on health behaviour and its role in health promotion was held in Pitlochry, Scotland in 1986. Technical support and financial assistance to this symposium were also provided by the Research Unit in Health and Behavioural Change, University of Edinburgh and the Economic and Social Research Council, London. The contributions made by some of the wide range of international experts at the symposium form the basis for the papers in this book.

One of the main aims of the symposium was to stimulate research into health beliefs and health behaviours at local, national, and international levels to help in the achievement of Health for All by the Year 2000. We hope that publication of this book will contribute significantly to this goal.

We wish to take this opportunity to acknowledge the help given by the many people involved in the planning and organizing of the Pitlochry Symposium and in the production of this book. In particular thanks go to the staff of RUHBC, and in particular Ms Jane Hopton for her work in relation to the final manuscript.

1987

R. A.
J. K. D.
I. K.
D. V. M.
J. T.

Contents

SECTION F
Discussion papers on a new agenda for research in health behaviour

Contributors

Zoltán Ajkay
Hungarian Institute for Pulmonology, Budapest, Hungary

Robert Anderson
Institute for Social Studies in Medical Care, London, United Kingdom

David Armstrong
Guy's Hospital Medical School, London, United Kingdom

John Ashton
Department of Community Health, University of Liverpool, Liverpool, United Kingdom

Ilona Bognár
Ministry of Health, Budapest, Hungary

Lamberto Briziarelli
Department of Hygiene, Experimental Centre for Health Education, University of Perugia, Italy

John K. Davies
Scottish Health Education Group, Edinburgh, United Kingdom

Kathryn Dean
Institute of Social Medicine, Copenhagen, Denmark

Pierpaolo Donati
Department of Sociology, University of Bologna, Bologna, Italy

Gary Hogelin
Center for Health Promotion and Education, Centers for Disease Control, Atlanta, USA

Esko Kalimo
Research Institute for Social Security, Social Insurance Institution, Helsinki, Finland

Ilona Kickbusch
World Health Organization Regional Office for Europe, Copenhagen, Denmark

Mihály Kökény
Office of the Government, Budapest, Hungary

Una Maclean
Department of Community Medicine, University of Edinburgh, Edinburgh, United Kingdom

David V. McQueen
Research Unit in Health and Behavioural Change, University of Edinburgh, Edinburgh, United Kingdom

Rose Martinez
Department of Health and Social Welfare, Madrid, Spain

Horst Noack
Institute for Social and Preventive Medicine, University of Berne, Berne, Switzerland

Don Nutbeam
Health Promotion Authority for Wales, Cardiff, United Kingdom

Janine Pierret
CERMES (Research Centre in Medical Illness and Social Science), Paris, France

Roisin Pill
Department of General Practice, University of Wales College of Medicine, Cardiff, United Kingdom

Ossi Rahkonen
Department of Public Health, University of Helsinki, Helsinki, Finland

Arja Rimpelä
Department of Public Health, University of Helsinki, Helsinki, Finland

Matti Rimpelä
Department of Public Health, University of Helsinki, Helsinki, Finland

Irving Rootman
Health Promotion Directorate, Canadian Ministry of Health, Ottawa, Canada

M. Stacey
Department of Sociology, University of Warwick, Coventry, United Kingdom

Juha Teperi
Department of Public Health, University of Helsinki, Helsinki, Finland

Armando Peruga
Department of Health and Social Welfare, Madrid, Spain

1

Introduction

ILONA KICKBUSCH

'The stage is set for a new public health revolution'
Lester Breslow, 1985

This brief introduction outlines some elements of a research agenda for health behaviour research in relation to health promotion. I hope to indicate how a new type of health behaviour research would assist in developing a clear theoretical and conceptual base for health promotion and a grounding of the issues researched in the realities of people's everyday lives.

The ecological and social understanding of health: the conceptual base of health promotion

Health promotion is based on a broad understanding of 'health' as the extent to which an individual or group is able, on the one hand, to realize aspirations and satisfy needs; and, on the other hand, to change or cope with the environment. This reaffirms the WHO definition of health, approved by Member States in 1948, reiterating that health goes beyond the absence of disease but adding a dynamic and process-based dimension. Health—as defined by WHO—is based on an understanding of public health that encompasses the notion of social responsibility for health: the components of physical and mental well-being need a foundation in a secure society. But it was not until the end of the 1970s—with the Declaration of Alma-Ata—that the importance of the social component of the WHO definition of health truly began to emerge and gain prominence and that the notion of 'social well-being' moved to the foreground. While this approach was developed in the light of current tools and knowledge on social factors in health, it poses at the same time a major challenge to the social science research community.

Socio-economic factors and social class differences constitute only the beginning of an in-depth understanding of people's way of life and health. In the light of our present-day knowledge, we extend social well-being to include components of the social environment such as cultural dynamics and social change, social support, and social relationships. Here lies the challenge to develop new types of research on health behaviour based on an ecological model of health that sees the individual as an integral part of a social group and acknowledges the biological as well as the non-biological components of health. In such a perspective health is a multi-dimensional phenomenon; the interaction between individuals and their social and physical environment is understood as integrated and holistic.

Health is also seen as a process reflecting activity and change with an implicit potential for enhancement rather than a static endpoint or product. It reflects a pattern of fluctuations, self-transformations, and self-transcendence involving crises and transitions. This makes it impossible always to draw clear lines between health and illness or to see health and illness as opposites of a continuum.

But health is more than its components: it is held together by spiritual and emotional notions of well-being, by perceptions of self and one's relationship to others.

If we aim to trace the major elements of an ecological and social model of health, we can state the following.

- It is concerned with the 'whole person, mind and body, one of a body, one of a family, and a member of society and culture. The social model recognizes the multiple interactions of these, and emphasizes well-being, fulfilment, independence, functioning in society, and social roles'. It is comprehensive and 'positive'.
- It is concerned with the social distribution of health, for example in relation to income, gender, age, education. It is aware that lifestyles reflect life changes.
- It aims at understanding cultural and personal meanings attached to health. For many people, health is not the highest goal in life. Health norms are often in conflict with a more important goal, be it happiness, adventure, or pure necessity. The large variations in health and illness behaviour from one culture to another show how many of the beliefs and behaviours related to health are learned within a specific cultural and social context.
- It takes into account the role of perceptions and emotions related to health. The subjective interpretation of health arises as a central focus of research and action.
- It aims at understanding health actions in the context of patterns of everyday life. People do not live as 'smokers', 'alcoholics', 'disabled', etc., but as whole people. It is a fact of everyday life that people must take risks, especially for people already living in restricted or deprived conditions. Health must not be used as an instrument for controlling social life.
- It implies a non-professional construction of health. It is becoming increasingly clear that health is not just a matter between doctors and patients. It is a total resource. Several decades of research now make it clear that most health maintenance and care is delivered by the people themselves.

- It sees self-reliance as an expression of human dignity and development. Self-care is the first form of care—and all other levels of professional care (also of professional primary health care) are supplementary and supportive.
- It implies that there is more than just one form of caring, curing, or healing. In every society, even those most dominated by a medical, professional model of health, we find many different forms of health care provision, and very often we find that the 'patients' move between several of these systems. It is important to note the continuous interaction between the three sectors of care, in relation to both knowledge and technical resources.

This ecological understanding of health, which clearly places the individual within a social, cultural, and physical environment, is the central conceptual base for health promotion. While the risk-factor prevention approach aims at establishing causal relationships between isolated factors and behaviours, the ecological promotion approach aims at identifying patterns of interaction between biological, personal, social, and environmental factors. It aims at enabling intervention based on the common life situations and/or life chances of certain groups rather than on intervention aimed at specific diseases. The patterns evolving from the interaction between the structural and the personal can be analysed in terms of 'health cultures'. The analysis of health therefore becomes concerned with a complexity of causes and outcomes, and aims at tracing their interaction.

This volume is intended to contribute towards such a wider understanding, and to point towards a new agenda for health behaviour research.

SECTION A
The development of concepts and research in health behaviour

INTRODUCTION

David V. McQueen

Clio would find little comfort in the extant histories of public health. Further, if that history were reviewed for insight into the development of concepts and research in health behaviour, there would be relatively little to report. Because of this historical vacuum the following chapters by Armstrong and Anderson should be seen as preliminary, but none the less as pioneering, efforts to develop an historical perspective on our field of research. They have provided two personal views of the history of health behaviour as a concept and Anderson has added a concern with the application of behavioural science research in public health.

Armstrong traces the historical background of the concept of health behaviour from its earlier development to what he sees as its emergence as a conceptual field in the 1960s. He focuses on the role of the body in relationship to the environment and how this role was slowly transferred from an emphasis on personal hygiene in public health to one of a psychological concern with conduct. Following a period, largely in the inter-war years, of involvement with mental hygiene combined with increasing development of morbidity surveys, much of the background for a 'new' science of health behaviour was well established. The 'science' of health behaviour began to flourish in the post-war period with new questions concerning the public's attitudes towards medical innovations. Notably, the issue was focused around how to stimulate the public's participation into an acceptable medical response by utilizing social science. The 1960s witnessed the flowering of interest with notions such as 'illness behaviour', and it was only after some time that health-related behaviours were partially freed from the underlying biomedical bias. Armstrong concludes with a personal view that current views of health behaviour leading to a 'new public health' may well be both 'liberating and repressive'.

Anderson picks up the research on health behaviour in the 1960s and reviews its development to the present time. The chapter reveals the richness of research in the area and traces the emergence of a research paradigm somewhat freed from a biological and disease model. None the less, his work points to the relative paucity of theory behind the emerging trends in health behaviour research. The material he reviews well illustrates the fundamental point that attempts at categorization of behaviour and an analytic approach tend to separate behaviour into conceptual pieces or fragments. What remains clear is that the search for an integrating theory of health behaviour is still wanting.

2

Historical origins of health behaviour

DAVID ARMSTRONG

Abstract

This chapter identifies three fundamental changes between the end of the nineteenth century and 1966 which enabled the term 'health promotion' to join the conceptual currency of our time.

There was a theoretical reconstruction of the field of health and illness. While much of clinical medicine continued within the framework of a binary and physical classification, public health underwent a profound reorganization during the twentieth century. By the inter-war years health was no longer construed as a nominal category in a binary classification but as a continuum. In other words, health was not fixed as the opposite of illness, but was something that could be improved or damaged by small degrees. Also, the conceptual space in which health and illness were located was transformed from the physical relationship of body and environment in nineteenth-century public health to the social matrix of bodies characterized by psycho-social attributes.

There were changes in the role identity of patients. The new perception of health and illness as existing in social spaces brought about two important changes in the identity of the patient: illness was not simply a physical object existing within the patient but patient subjectivity itself was a component of illness, and secondly patients were recruited as active monitors and actors with regard to their own bodies. Thus the patient became both object and subject of medicine.

A conceptual field emerged for comprehending the problem of behaviour. The early twentieth century world of instincts, conduct and habits was transformed into one of attitudes and behaviour. These newly-perceived attributes of people were essentially changeable and created scope for new health technologies such as health education, mental hygiene and health behaviour.

Introduction

In the nineteenth century there were two great systems of medical classification/management, namely clinical medicine and public health (Foucault 1977). Clinical medicine was essentially a binary system concerned with separating the healthy from the diseased. This separation was embodied in the theoretical distinction between the normal and the abnormal—that is, between the physiological and the pathological—the presence or absence of a fixed organic lesion within the body; it was reflected in practical techniques of segregation which, through the clinical examination and the process of diagnosis, enabled person to be separated from patient; and it showed itself in the increasing dominance of the hospital—which exiled the ill from the well—in the provision of health care.

Clinical medicine conceptualized illness as a localized pathological lesion but in contrast public health focused on a more abstract notion of disease which was contained in the movement of dirt in and out of bodies. Its domain of investigation was therefore not the body itself but the interface between the body and the environment, a sanitary space which carried the risk of dirt and contamination; and its diagnostic tool was not the stethoscope but the map, which enabled the spatial distributions of disease to be registered and plotted. Thus, whereas clinical medicine worked theoretically and practically on the basis of separating the healthy from the diseased, public health employed a system of constant monitoring and surveillance to safeguard the health of an entire population.

The binary clinical system of 'exile-enclosure', which separated the abnormal from the normal, constituted the dominant medical classification of the nineteenth and, indeed, twentieth centuries. But it was the public health system of multiple partitioning of a population and the surveillance of everyone which provided the origins and exemplar for twentieth-century developments in hygiene, health education and health behaviour.

The transformation of hygiene

Nineteenth-century public health was concerned with the physical interface between the body and the 'natural' environment of soils, climate, and habitations. Various substances—water, air, food, excreta—which passed between the body and environment were viewed as potentially dangerous, as possibly being contaminated by dirt. Public health therefore deployed a system of hygiene based on sanitation through which the interface between the body and the natural environment was constantly monitored, guarded and cleansed so as to prevent the transmission of disease across body boundaries.

At the beginning of the twentieth century a major shift occurred in the focus of public health. Instead of monitoring the space between the body and the environment, the new hygiene was concerned with the actual physical space between bodies themselves. Tuberculosis, for example, had been a disease of physical environment, of dirt, poor housing, and sanitation; in the early twentieth century it became a disease of social contact, of breathing, spitting, proximities. But the space between bodies not only had physical characteristics, it also had social. It was therefore only a small step for the physical space between bodies to be redefined as an essentially 'social' one and the possibility of a 'social medicine' to emerge (Armstrong 1983).

The space between bodies still possessed physical properties but it was the relationship of the bodies themselves which determined the health risk. Sanitation was therefore transformed from a scrutiny of the physical space between bodies and environment to the new techniques of a personal hygiene of the body. 'The old public health was concerned with the environment;' noted Hill in 1916, 'the new is concerned with the individual' (Hill 1916). The potentially active patient was beginning to present itself to medical perception.

Traditional clinical medicine involved an interaction between clinician and pathological lesion. The patient, as a person, had only existed within this dyad as a repository or, at most, rather unreliable translator for the lesion. Equally in nineteenth-century public health, the individual was little more than the physical matter through which disease passed in its movement from and between natural environments. For all branches of nineteenth-century medicine, therefore, the patient was no more than a passive physical object.

In the new public health, however, which stressed the importance of both physical and social relationships between bodies, the individual was consti-tuted as a more active physical and social being. Personal hygiene addressed this individual because it required commitment to certain activities, particu-larly those involving the sanitization of body interfaces such as skin, mouth, eyes, ears, teeth, bowels, etc., lest disease be transmitted from one person to another (e.g. Bigger 1937). In effect the object of the new personal hygiene was not the organic lesion but some activities of its potential host.

The reconstruction of patient identity through the new public health towards a more active and acting object, however, was only one part of this transformation in medicine. The other component of the new personal hygiene was the recruitment of the patient to the medical enterprise. In the nineteenth century the public official alone could monitor and control the dangers of natural environment; given the scope of the new hygiene, however, it could not rely on public health officials as its agents of surveil-lance, instead it demanded involvement of 'patients' themselves. If human bodies were to be monitored and sanitized medicine required the active co-operation of those same bodies: patients therefore had to be enlisted to practice their own hygienic regime; patients had to become agents of medicine, their own self-practitioners.

Thus the two related features of modern social medicine were forged early in the twentieth century. On the one hand, the patient as a person became the *object* of medical attention, particularly in his or her own actions. On the other hand, the patient was also the *subject* of medicine in the sense that patients were recruited to monitor their own bodies. Since then these two (and often confused) facets of patient identity have been explored, developed, and reinforced. The active body of the patient required study, guidance and control if illness was to be avoided and health achieved. The malleable subjective mind of the patient in its turn demanded education and training if it was successfully to monitor and bring under some control its otherwise capricious body.

The movement of bodies

Early in the twentieth century the concept of health behaviour as such had no existence. Indeed while the problem of behaviour was to achieve some limited recognition in 'behaviourism', most of the new discipline of psychology was concerned with the subject of human 'conduct' which was held to be the 'highest type of behaviour'. The term behaviour itself was reserved to describe 'certain peculiarities which are only found in the movement of living things' (McDougall 1908).

Although the new personal hygiene did not directly address the problem of behaviour it certainly implied some 'healthy' body movements. However, no formal conceptual link was forged between physical movement—perhaps the most rudimentary manifestation of behaviour—and health. Such a link was in fact first made by the new elementary schools which emerged at the end of the nineteenth century.

Universal primary education had the task of managing and transforming the body of the child. To accomplish this goal the new schools at first simply borrowed the same techniques which had evolved in the army to transform raw recruits into disciplined soldiers. Drill routines, 'marching, counter-marching, diagonal marching, changing ranks and so on' (Atkins 1904, p. 36) were initially popular. Later, with criticism of both the latent militarism in these exercises and of their tendency to produce a stiff body, more 'carefully graduated and scientifically calculated' movements were introduced (Atkins 1904, p. 151).

The disciplining of bodily movement in both army and school was gradually widened from the rigidity of drill to the more generalized techniques of physical training and physical education. The individual body could be trained, particularly through repetitive actions—so inculcating 'habits'—to achieve some goal such as fitness and efficiency. Training took control over the general physical development of the child, ensuring that full physical capacity was achieved (Newton 1907) and it also had a 'corrective effect' remedying or adjusting 'any obvious defects or incorrect attitude or action of the body, or any of its parts' (Board of Education 1909, p. 3).

But it was not only the drill sergeant and the teacher who trained the child's body but also the child itself: training could equally well—and undoubtedly more efficiently and permanently—be achieved through education. Pure training only worked at the level of habit forming: 'the child unconsciously acquires habits of discipline and order, and learns to respond cheerfully and promptly to the word of command' (Board of Education 1909, p. 5). Yet the more valuable aim was to instill the word of command into the child so it could function as its own drill master. 'Physical fitness should not be advocated by the teacher as an end in itself,' cautioned the English Board of Education in 1928, 'but as a means to promote the mental and moral health and character of the child' (Board of Education 1928).

Health behaviour in its most abstracted yet perhaps most fundamental form is represented by the physical movement of the body. The discovery of the elementary school was that behaviour as represented by physical activity could be fashioned and goal-directed. Posture, fitness and efficiency were the initial objectives but with the gradual extension of the techniques through which the body was manipulated—physical culture, sports, gymnastics, dance, exercises, and athletics—the goal widened towards a regime of total health.

Mental hygiene

In the nineteenth century the mind had been seen as located in the cerebral tissues. Its only pathology was insanity which was, in the main, inherited. In the twentieth century the mind, as conceptualized by the new discipline of psychology, was construed as something separate from the brain and instead linked to the new problems of personal relationships and coping. Whereas previously a few people, because of their heredity, were mentally at risk, in the twentieth century everybody was (Treadway 1936). New diseases emerged under the umbrella of the 'neuroses' and, as with training of the body, the child was seen to be particularly at risk. Twentieth-century medicine discovered the nervous child, the delicate child, the neuropathic child, the solitary child, the unstable child and the difficult child. Yet how could the mind be influenced by techniques of hygiene? The answer was through the body.

The link between mind and body was a complex one. On the one hand movement of the body had its effects on the mind: exercises could inculcate habits and, moreover, it seemed that the discipline of movement could focus the mind on the task in hand, eliminating stray thoughts—perhaps of a sexual nature—and build up 'character' (Hussey 1928). But equally, movement in some way reflected mental functioning. There was apparently 'a very close relationship between intelligence and success in athletics' (Ruble 1928), and mental problems might be expressed in poor movement co-ordination just as true character could be read from the sports field, the gymnasium, the athletics ground, and the dance school (Campbell 1940). Then, as now, exercise as a form of health behaviour was as much directed to the mind as to the body.

A strategy of 'mental hygiene' was advocated in the inter-war years to promote stable mental development. In the school, mental hygiene could prepare the citizens of tomorrow (Dicks 1948). Industry could be more efficient with due attention to the mental state of the worker as shown by industrial hygiene and the new human relations school of factory management. Illicit sexual thoughts which led to promiscuity and syphillis could, in their turn, be combated by 'social hygiene'.

The new techniques of mental surveillance, just as those of physical training, shifted the medical management of populations from a system of binary division to one of multiple partitioning. Health was not present or absent, it was graded. The healthy could become more healthy or less healthy. In the early drill routines in schools pupils were ordered in terms of size ('in succession, shortest on the right of the class, tallest on the left'—Interdepartmental Committee 1904, p. 17), in the classroom they were ordered in terms of Binet's system of IQ gradings, on the athletics field they were ranked according to speed, skill or prowess. Health and illness as fixed external referents continued in use within the medical sector—particularly the hospital—but elsewhere they began to lose their meaning. If, as the Peckham Health Centre reported in the 1930s, 93 per cent of the population had an identifiable pathology, what value a simple binary system for the management and ordering of populations? (Pearse and Crocker 1943).

In 1923 a collaborative venture between the city of Fargo in North Dakota and the Commonwealth Fund was inaugurated with the object of incorporating child health services into the permanent programme of the health department and public school system. An essential component of this plan was the introduction of health education in Fargo's schools, supervised by Maud Brown. Brown's campaign was, she wrote, 'an attempt to secure the instant adoption by every child of a completely adequate program of health behaviour' (Brown 1929, p. 2).

Prior to 1923 the state had required that elements of personal hygiene be taught in Fargo's schools 'but there was no other deliberately planned link between the study of physical well-being and the realization of physical well-being' (Brown 1929, p. 7). The Commonwealth Fund project had a two-pronged strategy. While the classroom was the focus for a systematic campaign of health behaviour, a periodic medical and dental examination both justified and monitored the educational intervention. In effect 'health teaching, health supervision and their effective co-ordination' were linked together. In Fargo 'health teaching departed from the hygiene textbook, and after a vitalizing change, found its way back to the textbook' (Brown 1929, p. 7). Fargo, however, did not mark the beginning of this change but rather its formalization: the old hygiene which had monitored the natural environment was replaced by various techniques which operated as integral parts of a surveillance machinery.

In his advice of 1919 on public education in hygiene Newman had commended the practice of hygiene, teaching of mothercraft, physical education and open-air education (Newman 1919). Fargo, from its insistence on four hours of physical exercises a day—two of them outdoors—to its concern with the mental maturation of the child, represented the realization of a new public health dream.

Towards a new public health

Fargo was a special instance of what could be achieved if the necessary public health resources and political will could be directed to a whole community. But for the proponents of the new personal hygiene, knowledge of the health of the population was uncertain. In the new regime health was continuously distributed and by and large techniques with which to measure such gradations were lacking. The only comprehensive records were those on mortality which represented the logic of a binary system. Certain diseases were notifiable but under-reporting was known to be common; some industrial sickness records were available but they related only to sickness causing absence from work; equally the rare attempt to measure all sickness had excluded those illnesses not attended by a doctor.

In the inter-war years interest grew in morbidity surveys which might better indicate the subtle health gradations between people. Where full health examinations were carried out—particularly amongst groups of school children—many 'correctable' defects were identified. Similarly, it was held that health examination of adults would enable the identification and treatment of incipient disease (Collins 1934). But health examinations by doctors were impractical in terms of resources and difficult in terms of technique (Britten 1931). More valuable were patient surveys such as the 9000 family periodic health canvas in the USA (Collins 1933). Such survey techniques eschewed the binary approach of clinical medicine which simply identified the diseased and separated them from the healthy; instead the survey established a continuity, a range of variations. Some clearly required immediate treatment. For others 'early attention to minor diversions from the normal may be means of preventing the development of serious disease' (Collins 1934). And also of course the apparently normal and healthy required instruction in the ways of healthy living so as to avoid even the slightest sign of impending non-health.

Public health in the 1930s established health as a precarious state, not simply the absence of disease. Such a view was furthered and consolidated in the famous 1952 WHO definition of health and the post-war concept of 'at risk', which effectively transposed health from being a state to being a goal. In part the new vision was still articulated on the early twentieth-century social problems of tuberculosis and venereal disease—both of which had been reconstructed into diseases of social conduct—but gradually the model and techniques of health they embodied were generalized across the full range of illness.

Some indication of the success of the new paradigm can be established from the questions addressed to the information service of the US Public Health Service. In an analysis of 10 000 'recent questions' in 1939, Oleson reported that 'in general, these figures indicate a shift in emphasis from consideration of disease as entities to those involving hygiene, sanitation, facilities for medical care, climate, diet and the like' (Oleson 1939, p. 769). In sum it had 'become obvious that the most effective way of safeguarding health is through personal effort'.

The war created the conditions for the new public health further to establish itself. Industrial hygiene to maximize production, mental hygiene to cope with 'physical and nervous strains' ('and toughen up America'). social hygiene to combat the problem of venereal disease ('scourge of armies and families') and campaigns finally to vanquish tuberculosis, all pointed the way towards a new approach to health (Shepherd 1941, p. 1356).

By the end of the war health education was firmly established as an essential part of the public health programme. 'Health authorities', wrote Derryberry in 1945, 'are becoming increasingly aware that many diseases are uncontrollable without the active participation of the people themselves' (Derryberry 1945). Whereas a few decades earlier the community was involved in public health only in so far as their electoral or political support was required, now people had to be involved from the very beginning of any programme because they themselves were the agents of health practice (Derryberry 1949).

Post-war reconstruction

Before the Second World War public health had been concerned with non-participation only to the extent that certain patients 'defaulted' from treatment, particularly from that of venereal disease. Another point for the articulation of ideas on patient behaviour emerged in April 1955 in the USA when the Salk vaccine was declared safe and an effective protection against poliomyelitis. A national vaccination programme commenced at once and became the new focus for the problems of participation within the public health literature. Here for once was a programme with undeniable benefits yet which the public failed to support wholeheartedly.

What were the public's attitudes towards vaccination? What factors precluded their involvement? Indeed the questions began even before the vaccine was proved to be safe and effective. As Clausen and his colleagues noted in their report on parental reactions to the vaccine in the trials, they 'may be useful in indicating in somewhat greater detail than is usually available the factors influencing participation in such a program and the attitude and characteristics of participants and non-participants' (Clausen *et al.* 1954, p. 1526). In short it was not so much that the study of participation would indicate the problem of poliomyelitis vaccination, but that the vaccination programme could be used to illuminate the whole issue of participation. 'Using the technics of social science research, it would seem fruitful to investigate further the methods of reaching and influencing those segments of the population which tend to be non-participants in such public health programs' (Clausen *et al.* 1954, p. 1536).

In similar fashion, response to community X-ray programmes for tuberculosis and to the new multi-phasic screening programmes focused attention on public participation (Hochbaum 1956, p. 377). But how was participation and non-participation to be explained? The first step was the discovery of culture. The old view, that as 100 per cent of Americans were of old stock, there were no cultural factors involved was wrong: 'obviously, culture is here as well as in Bali, if only we can see it around us' (Wishik 1958, p. 139). Thus 'a person's motivations are compounded out of his previous personal experiences and the cultural background from which he derives and in which he moves' (Wishik 1958). Whereas during the early part of the century human behaviour had seemed to be governed by instinct, that is from a fixed biological point, during the late 1950s public health discovered beliefs as the mainspring of human action. The theories of Rosenstock and his colleagues of why people failed to seek polio vaccination (Rosenstock *et al.* 1959) had become, by 1965, the basis for a more generalized model of health beliefs and focus on patient activity (Rosenstock 1965).

One of the effects of the recruitment of the patient as an integral component of health management was the change in the status and nature of 'patient' identity. The boundary between healthy person and patient became problematic. In the past the transition from person status to patient status had been marked by 'coming under the doctor'. In the new regime which made the patient both an object of medicine and a lay health practitioner, patienthood began to lose its old meaning. This shift was marked by the extension of patient status (or at least potential status) as everyone came under medical/health surveillance through the gradual recruitment of everyone to the medical enterprise. Post-war surveys of population morbidity and symptom prevalence confirmed that a rigid distinction between health and illness was meaningless: everyone had health problems, everyone was 'at risk', health care merely touched the tip of the morbidity iceberg (Last 1963). In addition the now problematic boundary between person and patient was subjected to a close analysis in the new subject of 'illness behaviour'.

Illness behaviour, a term invented by Mechanic in 1960 (Mechanic and Volkart 1960), has often been challenged (such as in Kasl and Cobb's classic paper of 1966) as too restricted, and failing to encapsulate the wider concerns of health behaviour. Yet illness behaviour was not only an explanation of certain health-related activities but also part of the post-war fascination with the weakening person–patient interface. The concept of illness behaviour showed that the transition between health and illness, person and patient was not predicated on an absolute and biological difference, but was underpinned by the notion of a person as their own health practitioner making judgements and decisions on the nature and boundaries of health and illness.

The patient was inseparable from the person because all persons had become patients, and with it changed their identity. Until the post-war years behaviour had been relatively unchangeable, set by heredity and repetitive patterning. In the post-war years behaviour became contingent: social psychologists, for example, discovered attitudes with which to replace instincts as one of the prime determinants of behaviour, the patient thus becoming a more unpredictable and variable being.

Perhaps the date of this transformation of patienthood can be established from the sudden interest in the placebo effect from about 1948 (Shapiro 1960). Before World War II the placebo effect went unnoticed: how could it possibly be identified in patients who functioned as passive robots? The recognition of the placebo effect signified the moment when subjective mental processes began to seize control of the body. Yet the 'discovery' of the placebo response not only reflected the post-war interest in the patient's mind, but also continued a process from earlier in the century when the patient had begun to be recruited to the medical enterprise through the spread of personal hygiene. Patient thought and deed, both consciously through personal hygiene and often unconsciously through the placebo, had an effect on health.

Medicine invented the placebo to describe this new patient role; it also discovered the doctor–patient relationship as a new and problematic topic (Armstrong 1982). The relationship was not only between practitioner and body as of old, but also between practitioner and subjective mind and between medical practitioner and quasi-medical practitioner. The doctor consulted as much with his patient as an 'agent' as with his patient as a body.

The old doctor–patient relationship—unreflective as it was—was constituted around a biological lesion in the patient's body. The medical task was diagnosis which directed attention to cause and treatment. Disease existed or it did not, diagnosis functioned to separate health from illness. But when health and illness lost their distinctiveness, when health became a continuum, the fundamental structure of medical knowledge changed. A binary system of diagnosis was essentially underpinned by a unimodal theory of aetiology in that only one factor need be present or absent to explain group membership. A system of health based on multiple partitioning required aetiology to be

something more extensive: thus medicine discovered multi-factorial aetiology in the post-war years which in its turn furthered the conceptual development of the field of health behaviours.

Just as the demise of a binary system of health produced multi-causal
models of illness, so the endorsement of incrementalist models of health
emphasized both the temporal characteristics of illness and the importance
of wider psycho-social factors. Thus post-war medicine discovered 'chronic
illness' as a major morbidity group and the 'community' as a locus for illness
(Arney and Bergen 1984; Armstrong 1985), both of which provided important contexts for the application of theories of health behaviour.

Prevention, promotion, and education

In 1900 medicine was represented by the physician armed with tools for the
exploration of individual physical bodies; the patient was that body, essentially passive, involved only to the extent that it must respond to and report
the outward manifestations of the organic disease. Health was the state which
was gained or lost by the disappearance or appearance of the lesion.

In the new regime of public health, medicine is no longer represented by
the solitary figure of the physician, but by a vast network ranging from the
comprehensive health system to community and 'informal' care. The patient
is a member of this network of surveillance, a 'producer' of health through
health-protective behaviour (Harris and Guten 1979). The patient is also a
consumer, an object of this medical enterprise; but whereas in the nineteenth
century the patient existed only as a passive body, the patient is now
constituted as a psycho-social being whose every movement and gesture is
monitored, evaluated and recorded by a medical machine based on a new
ideology of health. The patient has become an object within biographical and
social space rather than within strictly anatomical boundaries and these
extended features of patienthood have received increasing attention
(Armstrong 1984).

And finally the dream of the new medicine has reformed the relationship
between health and illness. No longer polar opposites within a binary
classification, they have become inextricably linked within a great continuum of health. On the one hand health is contained in illness; the
disabled, the chronically sick, the dying and the diseased can promote their
health by appropriate health behaviour, enabling reactions and successful
coping. Equally the germ of illness is now contained in health. Health has
become a temporal trajectory containing the seeds of illness which,
nevertheless, can be countered by preventive action, health promotion and
healthy living.

The binary medicine of the clinic, of course, still remains and the continuum of health in many cases simply remains a dream of the new public

health. Yet the conflict between these two systems is apparent as attempts are made to comprehend one in terms of the other. (Much of the terminological confusion may arise from framing the questions of the new medicine in terms of the old: inasmuch as disease prevention and some of the new health strategies—such as health education or certain aspects of health behaviour—belong to the binary system then they are incommensurable with the new health approaches which are able to see health in illness and vice-versa.)

A history of health behaviour cannot be reduced to a history of progress and enlightenment as there is no constant referent or standard by which change can be evaluated. Health behaviour is not simply a new approach to a set of problems, as the problems themselves have been recast. The new medicine has redefined itself, the patient, and the nature of health, and thereby established the social existence of new phenomena.

A health behaviour approach therefore helps reconstitute the objects towards which it is directed. The active participating individual proceeds from behaving to acting—better to capture the voluntaristic element in human activity; illness moves further from the body of the patient to social spaces, to problems of coping and adjustment; and medical strategies shift from the pronouncements of experts towards 'informed choice', non-directive counselling and a non-judgemental health behaviour as the old referents finally disappear. Influencing, manipulating, transforming, the new public health of continuous surveillance is at once both liberating and repressive, a dream of enlightenment held in the grip of a spectre of total social control.

References

Armstrong, D. (1982). The doctor–patient relationship: 1930–1980. In *The problem of medical knowledge* (ed. P. Wright, and A. Treacher). Edinburgh University Press.

Armstrong, D. (1983). *Political anatomy of the body: medical knowledge in Britain in the 20th century*. Cambridge University Press.

Armstrong, D. (1984). The patient's view. *Social Science and Medicine* **18**, 737.

Armstrong, D. (1985). Space and time in British general practice. *Social Science and Medicine* **20**, 659.

Arney, W. R. and Bergen, B. I. (1984). *Medicine and the management of living*. Chicago University Press.

Atkins, J. B. (1904). *National physical training: an open debate*. Ibister, London.

Bigger, J. W. (1937). *Handbook of hygiene*. Ballière Tindall, London.

Board of Education (1909). *Suggestions for the consideration of teachers*. HMSO, London.

Board of Education (1928). *Handbook of suggestions on health education*. HMSO, London.

Britten, R. H. (1931). The physical examination as an instrument of research. *Public Health Reports* **49**, 1671.

Brown, M. A. (1929). *Teaching health in Fargo*. Commonwealth Fund, New York.

Campbell, R. B. (1940). The psychological aspect of physical education. *Edinburgh Medical Journal* **47**, 351.

Collins, S. D. (1933). Causes of illness in 9000 families based on nationwide periodic canvasses, 1928–31. *Public Health Reports* **48**, 283.

Collins, S. D. (1934). Frequency of health examinations in 9000 families based on nationwide periodic canvasses, 1928–1931. *Public Health Reports* **49**, 321.

Clausen, J. A. *et al*. (1954). Parent attitudes towards participation of their children in polio vaccine trials. *American Journal of Public Health* **44**, 1526.

Derryberry, M. (1945). Health education in the public health program. *Public Health Reports* **60**, 1401.

Derryberry, M. (1949). Health is everybody's business. *Public Health Reports* **64**, 1293.

Dicks, H. V. (1948). Principles of mental hygiene. In *Modern trends in psychological medicine*, ed. N. G. Harris. Butterworth, London.

Foucault, M. (1977). *Discipline and punish: the birth of the prison*. Allen Lane, London.

Harris, D. M. and Guten, S. (1979). Health protective behaviour an exploratory study. *Journal of Health and Social Behaviour* **20**, 17.

Hill, H. W. (1916). *The new public health*. Macmillan, New York.

Hochbaum, G. M. (1956). Why people seek diagnostic X-rays. *Public Health Reports* **71**, 377.

Hussey, M. M. (1928). Character education in athletics. *American Physical Education Review* **3**, 578.

Report of the *Interdepartmental Committee on physical deterioration* (1904). HMSO, London.

Kasl, S. V. and Cobb, S. (1966). Health behaviour, illness behaviour and sick role behaviour I. *Archives of Environmental Health* **2**, 246.

Last, J. M. (1963). The clinical iceberg. *Lancet* **2**, 28.

McDougall, W. (1908). *An introduction to social psychology*. Methuen, London.

Mechanic, D. and Volkart, E. H. (1960). Illness behaviour and medical diagnosis. *Journal of Health and Human Behaviour* **1**, 86.

Newman, G. (1919). *An outline of the practice of preventive medicine*. HMSO, London.

Newton, R. C. (1907). What should be the attitude of the profession towards the hygiene of school life? *Journal of the American Medical Association* **49**, 663.

Oleson, S. D. (1939). 'What people ask about health. *Public Health Reports* **54**, 765.

Pearse, I. H. and Crocker, L. H. (1943). *The Peckham experiment*. Allen and Unwin, London.

Rosenstock, I. M. (1965). Why people use health services. *Millbank Memorial Fund Quarterly* **44**, 94.

Rosenstock, I. M. *et al*. (1959). Why people fail to seek poliomyelitis vaccination. *Public Health Reports* **74**, 98.

Ruble, V. W. (1928). A psychological study of athletes. *American Physical Education Review* **33**, 216.

Shapiro, A. K. (1960). A contribution to the history of the placebo effect. *Behavioural Science* **5**, 109.

Shepherd, W. P. (1941). A national emergency exists. *Public Health Reports* **56**, 1351.

Treadway, W. L. (1936). The place of mental hygiene in a federal health program. *Public Health Reports* **51**, 181.

Wishik, G. M. (1958). Attitudes and reactions of the public to health programs. *American Journal of Public Health* **48**, 139.

3

The development of the concept of health behaviour and its application in recent research

ROBERT ANDERSON

Introduction

This chapter will pick up some threads from the previous chapter on the historical origins of concepts and practice in health behaviour. It will consider how researchers have responded to, and supported, changes in foci of interest from illness to health, and from the role of medicine to how people seek to promote their own health. Beginning in the middle of the 1960s, the chapter looks at developments in the conceptualization and modelling of health behaviour, and considers some of the results from research.

The burgeoning academic (not to mention commercial) literature on 'health behaviour' reflects a diversity of approaches: from aetiology and causal analysis, to assessment of interventions, identification of processes of change and towards the formulation of health policy. This variety and complexity of interests has drawn in researchers from several disciplines, who have identified their own niche or spectrum of research issues in health behaviour: anthropology and the nature of health beliefs, meanings of health, interpretations and evaluations of behaviours that characterize different cultural and social groups; epidemiology and the relationship between behaviours and habits and health status; sociology and the significance of gender, social class, family relations and the economy for health behaviour; psychology and the measurement of attitudes and concerns, motivations and images of health, mind and body.

There is a crude working distinction between research which takes health behaviour as the dependent or the independent variable; that is, between research which seeks to understand the development and maintenance of health behaviour, and that which seeks to explain something else—usually death, disease or future health behaviour, but it could be morale or life satisfaction, as determined in part by health behaviour. Most of this latter research, looking at health behaviour as the independent variable, has been developed as part of epidemiology, identifying risk factors for, and the social distribution of, specific diseases—this field is not covered in this chapter. However, results from these epidemiological studies which have dealt with general health outcomes (e.g. Benfante *et al*. 1985, and particularly the Alameda County Study—Belloc and Breslow 1972; and Wiley and Camacho 1980) are important since their measurement of health practices has had a profound influence on the conceptualization of the dependent variable in other studies.

Concepts of health behaviour

About ten years ago Dowie (1975) reviewed the field of research in health behaviour and argued that most of the existing literature had been dominated by an inappropriate, medical paradigm; concepts and the behaviours of interest were derived from a biological and disease model, as opposed to a social and health model. He and later authors reflected that this was associated with the dominance, in conceptual discussions, of the definition offered by Kasl and Cobb (1966). (It should be noted, however, that most authors employing the term 'health behaviour' did so without recourse to conceptual discussion; they used the concept as an umbrella to cover all and sundry behaviours related to health and illness.) The significance of Kasl and Cobb's formulation was that they distinguished health behaviour from illness and sick-role behaviours, and defined it as 'any activity undertaken by a person believing himself to be healthy for the purpose of preventing disease or detecting it at an asymptomatic stage' (Kasl and Cobb 1966, p. 246).

Although Kasl and Cobb defined health behaviour by the intentions of the person, most researchers seem to have interpreted this in terms of medically approved practices designed to prevent disease. Health behaviour became equivalent to preventive behaviour 'inasmuch as it consists of utilisation of health services for the assumed purpose of maintaining or improving one's health and avoiding the effects of illness' (Steele and McBroom 1972). The foci of most studies in the period up to ten years ago was on the use of preventive health services and factors influencing this—on people as 'consumers' of services rather than on how people sought to attain health as 'producers' of this commodity (Dowie 1975).

The omission from consideration of lay or self-defined health behaviour was being challenged in the United States during the early 1970s (Maklan *et al*. 1974) and is best known from studies which adopted the approach of Harris and Guten (1979). Typically, they investigate a range of self-defined (though not necessarily self-initiated) behaviours, labelled 'health protective behaviour' and defined as 'any behaviour performed by a person regardless of his or her perceived health status, in order to protect, promote or maintain his or her health, whether or not such behaviour is objectively effective towards that end.' (Harris and Guten 1979, p. 18). This conceptualization explicitly calls attention to individuals undertaking behaviours that they believe are protective, regardless of whether these beliefs correspond to professional medical advice. It also avoids the problematic distinction between symptomatic and asymptomatic individuals—a distinction that has occupied much social scientific research, exploring the conditions under which a given bodily state is viewed as symptomatic and results in a decision to seek medical help. Finally, Harris and Guten leave the meaning of health open to the individual, thus opening the door to consideration of mental and social aspects, as well as concepts of physical disease which seem to represent the horizons of earlier formulations.

The conceptualization of Harris and Guten does not distinguish between behaviours undertaken at the initiative of the individual or family from those carried out on the recommendation of a health professional. A more recent elaboration of the concept of health protective behaviour (Berkanovic 1982) has embraced this distinction, while also seeking to reintroduce the issue of symptoms. Berkanovic differentiates 'lifestyle changes' undertaken by asymptomatic individuals from 'treatments' which are defined as those undertaken by people with symptoms. He does not make clear how changes unrelated to the symptoms of people taking 'treatments' are classified. However, this approach comes close to defining health behaviour as self-care, and other authors have subsumed health behaviour within the broader concept of self-care (Hickey 1986). Perhaps 'health behaviour' like 'health promotion' has a current attractive fund-raising appeal; there appears to be a recent tendency to embrace health behaviour within another discipline or research area. In one review of health behaviour research for WHO, the author begins with . . . 'a definition which has received widespread acceptance . . . this definition stated that behavioural medicine as it was termed . . . (Sanson-Fisher 1984).

A significant feature of recent conceptualizations has been the disaggregation of 'health behaviour' into its constituents, distinguishing principally between behaviours intended to reduce the risk of disease or accident, and those intended more generally to improve health (e.g. Rakowski 1986); and, to a lesser extent, between medically approved (preventive) practices and self-defined health behaviours (e.g. Stott and Pill 1983). The tendency has been for 'preventive' and 'health promotive' behaviours to be defined on the basis of expert medical opinion, so that the individual may have both or neither purpose in mind when he or she engages in the behaviour.

Few conceptualizations (Maklan *et al.* 1974) explicitly discuss health behaviour as being directed at environmental as well as personal change, and none appear to include collective as well as individual behaviour. Considering, however, the 'grassroots' origin of much health promotion (Anderson 1984), it seems appropriate to consider health behaviour in lay-defined terms, covering not only what individuals do to or for themselves, and for their families but also their involvement in group or community activities, including those designed to promote a social or physical environment more conducive to health. The interests of different programmes and policies for health promotion will require analysis of the range of health-related be- haviours—positive, preventive and probably also health-endangering behaviour. At present researchers are working with a diversity of (often implicit) conceptualizations, but tend to focus on individual, self-oriented behaviour of the preventive or health-endangering kind. Their varying terms of reference have their parallel in the mixed systems for investigating health behaviour.

Operationalization

Inadequate specification of the concepts has led to the interchangeable use of terms such as health habits, health practices and health behaviour. Their operationalization has, if anything, been more consistent, generally in terms of either risk factors for specific diseases or as a selected range of medically approved preventive behaviours—contacts with health professionals for advice, immunizations or check-ups, and carrying out approved practices.

The selection of health practices often reflects those from the Alameda study (Belloc and Breslow 1972) or closely related everyday activities. Tapp and Goldenthal (1982) asked people for the frequency with which they engaged in behaviours clustered around eight categories: nutrition, tobacco use, alcohol use, drug use, road and water safety, exercise and physical activity, rest and relaxation, personal health care. For preventive health procedures, use of physical and dental examinations have typically been investigated, selected as actions that are assumed to represent the rational medical model (Steele and McBroom 1972). In their study of working-class women, Stott and Pill (1983) looked at 'health procedures' operationalized as participation in breast self-examination, cervical smear tests, visits to dentist for self and children and ante-natal visits.

In general, in these approaches, the researcher checks the individual's personal behaviour against whatever list of activities have been considered appropriate to represent protection of health. It is the researcher who defines the activities, so that 'the range and typology of health behaviour is limited only by the imagination of the researcher and the purposes of the research' (Steele and McBroom 1972, p. 383). Consensus on the importance of different behaviours is yet to be established, although, for a recent national survey in the United States (Harris *et al.* 1984), 103 health experts were interviewed and asked to rate the priority of each of 65 health and safety factors affecting adults and children. These ratings were used to develop a composite Prevention Index. The development of these indices and cumula- tive scores is a common goal, but one which many who have tried view with doubts because of problems with internal consistency and reliability of the measures (Seemen and Seemen 1983).

The selection of health behaviours has usually been determined by state-of-the-art understanding of the role of behaviour in the aetiology or avoidance of illness. However, judgements about what constitutes an appropriate level of different behaviours require technical knowledge which is often lacking or disputed (take exercise and use of alcohol as examples). The desire to count, to make number and frequency observations and recommendations may have led to more research in some areas than in others. It is easier to operationalize and ask about certain discrete behaviours, e.g. physician visits, number of cigarettes smoked, than to operationalize behaviours like information seeking, strategies for management of stress, or social participation. Some activities of everyday living have been reincarnated as 'health behaviours' in less research than sometimes seems the case, given the plethora of pronouncements on the 'healthy' life; it is difficult to do illuminating research in areas such as diet, exercise, and drinking.

Apart from those studies using open-response designs to identify behaviours or changes in behaviour that people undertake to protect or improve their health, there appears to have been little attempt to incorporate subjective intention or meaning into surveys of health behaviour. People have not usually been asked whether they moderate their drinking, indulge in excessive exercise, or abstain from smoking in order to maintain their health or for some other reason—although this makes significant differences to the results (Anderson 1983). The dominant research strategy appears to have been to document the frequencies of involvement in different (researcher-defined) health behaviour, and then to seek to understand patterns of behaviour by exploring the effects of a set of exploratory variables.

Most of the data have come from self-reports in surveys of a more (e.g. Danchik 1981) and less (e.g. Stott and Pill 1983) structured kind. Usually information has been derived from questions about specific preventive or health-promoting behaviours, and often very few behaviours have been considered. Information on other researcher-defined health behaviours has been found in other non-health surveys of food consumption, family expenditure, and leisure activities. Some analyses of trends or economic aspects of health behaviour are drawn from commercial data on sales of alcohol, tobacco, jogging shoes, and 'health foods'. There appears to have been little use of diary or observation techniques, although more ethnographic approaches have been used to investigate some of the 'exploratory' variables, such as health beliefs (Cornwell 1984), and to look at the social meaning of some behaviours, such as smoking (Graham 1976).

Results from research

Much of the previous discussion has drawn heavily upon accounts from the American literature or research looking at the determinants of medically approved behaviours, particularly the use of specific preventive health care services. This research has been extensively reviewed for both the US and the fewer UK studies (Blaxter 1981; Cartwright and O'Brien 1976; Anderson 1984)—it is not considered in detail here. However, the main explanatory variables for the use of preventive services (apart from the accessibility and availability of these services) have formed the basis for the exploration of health practices—socio-economic status, health beliefs, education, and social participation.

A substantial concern regarding the usefulness of a concept like health behaviour is whether in fact it represents a particular phenomenon with common determinants of its components, or whether the factors influencing the development of its elements are different. Harris and Guten (1979) reported that it was unreasonable to generalize from findings about preventive behaviour to other health practices. They found that family income and education were related to performance of both health practices and preventive care, but in opposite directions. In this and other studies which have asked people to define their health behaviour the use of health services is mentioned by only a small proportion of people, well behind behaviours linked to diet, exercise, and relaxation (Anderson 1984).

Harris and Guten (1979) concluded that 'people who obtain preventive examinations are no more or less likely to perform other types (of health protective behaviour) than are people who do not get them'. As in other studies (e.g. Maclean *et al*. 1984; Langlie 1977) the use of preventive services is associated with some health practices and not with others—the pattern is not consistent. In their recent study Stott and Pill (1983) reported some positive association between engaging in preventive procedures and health practices, but found little internal consistency in either measure. This literature points to the multi-dimensional nature of health behaviour—but the dimensions and how different behaviours cluster appears to be a function of which activities have been examined and how they have been measured. Tapp and Goldenthal (1982) examined the interrelationships of health behaviours, employing factor analysis to examine the dimensions of these behaviours, and interpreted three factors as reflecting: health promotion activities; avoidance of health risks; and a lack of awareness of good health practices. Harris and Guten (1979) identified five clusters of behaviours, while Langlie (1977), looking at the inter-correlations of 11 scales, found two distinct dimensions which she labelled 'direct risk' (e.g. driving, personal hygiene, smoking) and 'indirect risk' (e.g dental care, immunizations, exercise). The independent variables related to the two types of behaviour were distinctive, although age and sex were generally important.

Among the dimensions of health behaviour, the question arises as to whether any consistent pattern of interrelated behaviours can be identified. The responses appear quite modest: a few behaviours like not smoking and taking physical exercise seem to be associated (e.g. Mechanic 1979; Rimpela 1980), but there is little evidence of more extensive clustering of health-promoting behaviours. Perhaps because health-damaging behaviours have received more and more sophisticated attention, there is stronger evidence of some consistent clustering. Jessor (1982) concludes, from a review of research on adolescent behaviour, that there is substantial covariation in the use of cigarettes, alcohol and drugs that holds equally for males and females; furthermore, the different 'problem' behaviours all relate negatively to conventional behaviour such as involvement with the Church and school achievement. Considering the clustering of a more diverse range of risk behaviours among adults the interrelations seem weaker but still present. Kok *et al.* (1982) looked for the simultaneous occurrence of smoking, obesity, inadequate nutrition, and physical inactivity in a random sample of the Dutch adult population. They report that the behaviours did not cluster systematically but equally were not independent from one another. They compared adults with several and no risk factors, finding that men, those with low education and low occupation were disproportionately in the former group.

Doubts about the unidimensionality of health behaviour have not deterred researchers from devising cumulative scores of health practices, the best known of which is from the Alameda study and appears to have predictive validity (Wiley and Camacho 1980). More recently the Prevention Research Centre have deployed the Prevention Index (Harris *et al.* 1984) in a national survey showing that the practice of 'key preventive habits' was more common among women, those with higher incomes, in professional and managerial occupations, among those describing their health as better and among those who say they have 'a greater deal of control' over their future health. In both the Alameda and national studies, people aged 65 and over have consistently high scores—does this mean that they are more positively oriented to health promotion, or is it that they are a cohort of survivors, people whose social context does not encourage drinking alcohol, or just that they generally have too little money to be big consumers?

In the interests of research which has often had a practical focus, there has been a consistent search for those attitudes, beliefs or modifiable conditions which are associated with patterns of health behaviour. The results appear to have been generally disappointing: 'there appear to be few studies that can account for much variance in health protective behaviours through either mutable or immutable factors' (Berkanovic 1982, p. 235). The major

variables considered have been socio-demographic (education, employment, marital status), attitudes to health (beliefs, values, responsibility,
control) and social involvement (participation in clubs, church membership,
networks, social support). Many studies have found some relationship
between the variable of interest and the dependent variable, but most often
when this latter has been use of a preventive service (Seemen and Seemen
1983; King 1982; Langlie 1977; Jansen 1984). The most certain conclusion
seems to be that social networks, attitudes to health, and socio-demographic
characteristics all exert some influence on health behaviour, that they
interact, and that no single factor accounts for any major part of the variance.
Most likely, the variables are not consistent in the importance of their
influence on the different dimensions of health behaviour (Stott and Pill
1983).

Most of the research on health behaviour has been cross-sectional, asking
about attitudes and behaviour at the same time, and thus possibly exaggerat-
ing their association. Green *et al.* (1985) have looked for and suggested
reasons why this patterning does not often appear in practice—but they were
able to draw upon few studies which have examined the development,
maintenance and change of behaviours. In one study which investigated
positive health behaviours in childhood and sixteen years later most of the
findings were equivocal: Mechanic and Cleary (1980) reported little evidence of stability in behaviours over time, nor were they successful in
identifying factors which influenced the maintenance of positive health
behaviour.

Berkman (1982) has reviewed the literature on development of health
behaviours and identifies the significance of: typical ways of coping with
pressures and with tensions; the social acceptability of the behaviour; and the
influence of important individuals, such as parents or peers. However, nearly
all the evidence has accumulated from research on health-damaging behaviours; there is little information on the factors influencing the development
of health behaviours other than smoking, drinking, and use of preventive
services. Considering the multi-dimensionality of health behaviour and the
different factors associated with clusters in the cross-sectional studies there
seems reason to be cautious about Berkman's assertion that: 'While there is
certainly a dearth of information in this area there is also little reason to
suspect that other health practices which are common and not deviant
behaviours would not be associated with social and cultural factors in much
the same way as the above-mentioned practices (smoking and drinking)'
(Berkman 1982, p. 17).

Finally, on changing patterns of health behaviour, there is a lot of information about trends in some behaviours, particularly smoking, diet and
exercise, from periodic surveys by government and commerce. However,
there is little agreement about why some people change and others do not

(McDermott 1980). There has been interest in how changes in health behaviours may influence mortality from specific diseases (e.g. Beaglehole 1986) but much less in how changes in some behaviours may be linked to changes in other behaviours, and how the whole is related to changes in more positive aspects of health.

There is some indication from a retrospective study that younger people and those in higher social classes are more likely to change behaviour with the intention of improving their health (Berkanovic 1982); but another study, asking about a longer period of time, found no such difference (Anderson 1983)—perhaps reflecting a difference in the pace of health changes between the USA and the UK. Among the few studies of diffusion of health (preventive check-ups) practices, Ellenbogen *et al*. (1968) reported that among rural communities in upper New York State those who were least educated were least likely to take up the new services. In North Karelia, it appears that the initial diffusion of knowledge and ideas was to upper income and more highly educated groups, but that ultimately there were no uniform patterns associated with social structure (Vaskilampi 1981). Research on the diffusion of health behaviours, and understanding of the processes of change over time are little developed. For interpreting change over time using retrospective accounts, Anderson (1983) showed there was a need to consider the intention of the change, current health status and normal patterns of change in behaviour over the life cycle.

The contribution of research

Most research in this field has been ostensibly practical rather than theoretical—intended to identify factors which would indicate the means of changing people's behaviour. These means might be fiscal, legislative, community development, or organizational change, but the main beneficiary of the research is intended to be health promotion—in the community, in general practice, at the workplace, and in the mass media. Vaskilampi (1981) has shown how, in the North Karelia project, the methods and knowledge of the social sciences contributed to the emergence of a community health intervention programme. She notes that the definition of the goal of these programmes has generally been in disease terms, so that 'In health education, medical professionals define the values and norms of behaviour. Therefore, that which is healthy is good, and that which is unhealthy is bad. Thus the medical profession is an agent of social control in everyday life' (Vaskilampi 1981, p. 193). As debates continue about the objectives of health education and about its relationships to the priorities of medicine many will disagree with the sentiments here, but it appears as a reasonable general assessment of the purpose to which much of the work described as 'health behaviour' research has been put.

The general contribution of research has been conceived mainly in terms of planning and prediction, practice evaluation and policy development. So far most effort has been in understanding a range of medically-defined behaviours, almost all related to the avoidance of physical health problems, rather than to maintaining health in its broadest sense, including emotional and social aspects. Different behaviours and different underlying factors are likely to be more or less significant depending upon the outcome of interest. There is some concern that even in the most researched areas of use of preventive health services, relatively modest results only have been achieved in identifying variables which account for differences in patterns (see, for example, Coburn and Pope 1974; Dean 1984). This is not to say though that some variables are not related in a fairly constant way to some behaviours (e.g. social class and smoking rates, sex and use of alcohol, socio-economic status and use of preventive health services). Perhaps the most consistent relationships have been with social variables, which in principle offer prospects for targeting compensatory interventions to those least likely to take advantage of current opportunities. This raises questions though about the ethics as well as the effectiveness of measures aimed at changing the health orientations and knowledge of 'target' groups; that is, to ask to what extent are the preferences, priorities and prospects of target groups incorporated into health programmes, as well as to what extent do any combination of variables account for enough variance in health behaviour to warrant the cost of programmes aimed at changing them?

Some final observations

Many points have been made several times in different parts of this overview: that the main questions for research in health behaviour have been formulated by those concerned with the aetiology and prevention of diseases; that outcomes have been preoccupied with the body and its maintenance, and not with emotional or social dimensions of health; that there has been more interest in the use of preventive health services than in everyday health practices; that research has not been very successful in accounting for variation in health behaviour; that health behaviour is multi-dimensional and that it is not possible to generalize from factors related to one behaviour to factors related to another; and that factors investigated have reflected those which were potentially modifiable by health education rather than those which might respond to different patterns of workplace or community organization.

In considering these trends and priorities in previous research what are the implications for future development in relation to current ideas about health promotion? This concept seems to demand a broadening of approaches to investigate behaviours related to a more extensive concept of health, and, in particular, to look at 'positive health behaviours'. The focus has moved from disease to health, albeit without the conceptual clarity which would lead to operationalization of the behaviours of interest. However, it is clear that there will be an interest in those activities people engage in to promote their health which are social as well as individual. So, involvement in group activities to change the environment may be part of health behaviour as well as individual activities for and to oneself. The concept of health promotion emphasizes everyday choices for health and community involvement; it therefore seems appropriate that any concept of health behaviour should incorporate the lay-defined approach. The contribution of research in health behaviour to health promotion will be diverse and could be expanded by three related types of research study; on the social meaning of health behaviour; on explanatory variables through cross-sectional studies; and on analysis of change in behaviour through longitudinal studies.

Different social and cultural environments offer people varying frames of reference through which to view health behaviour and offer different standards for evaluating it. This may be related to different concepts of health and to different perceptions of the debits and benefits associated with health in comparison with other goals in life. It may be that for some groups health beliefs are weak predictors of health behaviours because it is only one—and often not the most important—value competing for the individual's time and energy. Understanding behaviours will demand knowledge of when people eat, drink or whatever, and with whom; how they view the intention of the behaviour, and what they perceive to be the relation between their everyday behaviour and health. This sort of information will provide a better basis for interpreting the results of surveys. The variables which might account for some of the gap between knowledge and behaviour continue to demand investigation in cross-sectional surveys. In so far as health promotion implies an interest in a broader range of positive and self-defined behaviour, there is a requirement for descriptive data to establish the relationship between these and other health practices or preventive activities. There will be many opportunities with this diversity of behaviours to look at their relationship to one another and to seek again to identify 'clusters' or dimensions of behaviour. However, the application of more sophisticated explanatory variables must be incorporated into models of development and change. The pattern of factors associated with maintenance of a behaviour may be different from the socialization or environmental factors associated with its development. And the identification of correlates or antecedents of health behaviour does not tell us 'how to change' that behaviour; if, for example, behaviour is associated with social support or health beliefs, that knowledge does not tell us how to change those beliefs or social norms; or precisely what the effects of changing these variables would be. From the point of view of translating research on health behaviour into the practices of health promotion, it seems appropriate to end with a quotation used by Jessor (1982):

'Sociologists may take comfort from trying to find out why things are as they are, rather than learning how things that are can be made different. But social policy is informed more by the latter than by the former.'

References

Anderson, R. (1983). How have people changed their health behaviour? *Health Education Journal* **42**, 82–6.

Anderson, R. (1984). Health promotion: an overview. *European Monographs in Health Education Research* **6**, 1–126.

Beaglehole, R. (1986). Medical management and the decline in mortality from coronary heart disease. *British Medical Journal* **292**, 33–5.

Belloc, N. B. and Breslow, L. (1972). Relationships of physical health status and health practices. *Preventive Medicine* **1**, 409–21.

Benfante, R., Reed, D., and Brody, J. (1985). Biological and social predictors of health. *Journal of Chronic Diseases* **38**, 385–95.

Berkanovic, E. (1982). Who engages in health protective behaviours? *International Quarterly of Community Health Education* **2**, 225–37.

Berkman, L. (1982). The social context of health behaviours. Paper to WHO meeting on lifestyles and living conditions and their impact on health. Hohr-Grenzhausen.

Blaxter, M. (1981). *The health of children: a review of research on the place of health in cycles of disadvantage*. Heinemann Educational, London.

Calnan, M. (1984). The health belief model and participation in programmes for the early detection of breast cancer. *Social Science and Medicine* **19**, 823–30.

Cartwright, A. and O'Brien, M. (1976). Social class variation in health care and in the nature of general practitioner consultations. In *The sociology of the NHS* ed. M. Stacey. Sociological Review Monograph 22, University of Keele, pp. 77–98.

Coburn, D. and Pope, C. (1974). Socioeconomic status and preventive health behaviour. *Journal of Health and Social Behaviour* **15**, 67–78.

Cornwell, J. (1984). *Hard-earned lives: accounts of health and illness from East London*. Tavistock, London.

Danchik, K. (1981). *Highlights from wave I of the national survey of personal health practices and consequences: United States 1979*. US Department of Health & Human Services. Publication No. (PHS) 81–1162.

Dean, K. (1984). Influence of health beliefs on lifestyles: what do we know? *European Monographs in Health Education Research* No. 6, 127–49.

Dowie, J. (1975). The portfolio approach to health behaviour. *Social Science and Medicine* **9**, 619–31.

Ellenbogen, B., Lowe G., and Danley, R. (1968). The diffusion of two preventive health practices. *Inquiry* **5**, 62–71.

Graham, H. (1976). Smoking in pregnancy; the attitudes of expectant mothers. *Social Science and Medicine* **10**, 399–405.

Green, L., Wilson, A., and Lovato, C. (1985). What changes can health promotion achieve and how long do these changes last? The trade-offs between expediency and durability. *Paper to HEC meeting*, Harrogate, England.

34 *Robert Anderson*

Harris, D. and Guten, S. (1979). Health-protective behaviour: an exploratory study. *Journal of Health and Social Behaviour* **20**, 17–29.

Harris, L. *et al.* (1984). *Prevention in America: steps people take—or fail to take—for better health*. Prevention Research Centre.

Hickey, T. (1986). Health behaviour and self-care in late life: an introduction. In *Self-Care and Health in Old Age*, ed. K. Dean, T. Hickey, and B. E. Holstein, pp. 1–11. Croom Helm, London.

Jansen, J. H. (1984). Participation in the first and second round of mass-screening for colorectal cancer. *Social Science and Medicine* **18**, 633–6.

Jessor, R. (1982). Critical issues in research on adolescent health. In *Promoting Adolescent Health*, pp. 447–65. Academic Press, London.

Kasl, S. and Cobb, S. (1966). Health behaviour, illness behaviour and sick-role behaviour. *Archives of Environmental Health* **12**, 246–66.

King, J. (1982). The impact of patients' perceptions of high blood pressure on attendance at screening: and extension of the Health Belief Model. *Social Science and Medicine* **16**, 1079–91.

Kok, F., Matroos, A., Van den Ban, A., and Hautvast, J. (1982). Characteristics of individuals with multiple behavioural risk factors for coronary heart disease: The Netherlands. *American Journal of Public Health* **72**, 986–91.

Langlie, J. (1977). Social networks, health beliefs and preventive health behaviour. *Journal of Health and Social Behaviour* **18**, 244–60.

McDermott, W. (1980). Medicine: the public's good and one's own. *World Health Forum* 123–32.

Maclean, U., Sinfield, D., Klein, S., and Harnden, B. (1984). Women who decline breast screening. *Journal of Epidemiology and Community Health* **38**, 278–83.

Maklan, C., Cannell, C. F., and French, J. P. R. (1974). Subjective and objective concepts of health: a back-ground statement for research. Michigan, Institute for Social Research.

Mechanic, D. (1979). The stability of health and illness behaviour: results from a 16-year follow-up. *American Journal of Public Health* **69**, 1142–5.

Mechanic, D. and Cleary, P. D. (1980). Factors associated with the maintenance of positive health behaviour. *Preventive Medicine* **9**, 805–14.

Rakowski, W. (1986). Preventive health behaviour and health maintainance practices of older adults. In *Self care and health in old age* (ed. K. Dean, T. Hickey, and B. E. Holstein), pp. 94–129. Croom Helm, London.

Rimpela, M. (1980). Incidence of smoking among Finnish youth—a follow-up study. Tampere, Kansanterveystieteen julkaisuya. M56/80.

Sanson-Fisher, R. (1984). *Health behaviour research in Australia, New Zealand and Papua New Guinea: an overview*. Prepared for WHO South Pacific Division.

Seemen, M. and Seemen, T. (1983). Health behaviour and personal autonomy: a longitudinal study of the sense of control in illness. *Journal of Health and Social Behaviour* **24**, 144–60.

Steele, J. and McBroom, W. (1972). Conceptual and empirical dimensions of health behaviour. *Journal of Health and Social Behaviour* **13**, 382–92.

Stott, N. and Pill, R. (1983). *A study of health beliefs, attitudes and behaviour among working class mothers*. Department of General Practice, Welsh National School of Medicine, Cardiff.

Tapp, J. and Goldenthal, P. (1982). A factor analytic study of health habits. *Preventive Medicine* **11**, 724–8.

Vaskilampi, T. (1981). Sociological aspects of community based health intervention programmes: the North Karelia project as an example. *Revue Epidemiologie et Sante Publique* **29**, 187–97.

Wiley, T. and Camacho, T. (1980). Lifestyle and future health: evidence from the Alameda County study. *Preventive Medicine* **9**, 1–21.

SECTION B
Approaches to the study of health behaviour

INTRODUCTION

Robert Anderson

Studies of health behaviour have been undertaken in several different research traditions, with different emphases depending in part upon the questions of interest as well as the methods of investigation that were available or preferred. So, making very crude distinctions, epidemiologists, for example, have typically considered a relatively narrow band of 'risk behaviours'—linking structured measurements of the frequencies and intensities of specific behaviours to disease outcomes. Social scientists, on the other hand, have been more engaged on the identification of factors associated with the development of different lifestyles. Within this group, there is a long-standing literature in social psychology on attitudes and knowledge associated with health behaviours, usually those considered deleterious to health. In the field of sociology, there has been considerable research on social and environmental conditions predisposing to different lifestyles. The various mediating variables related to cultural meanings and values have received less attention in European societies than in more 'exotic' cultures, but anthropologists have begun to look more seriously at their own societies to explore explanatory models and beliefs related to health as well as to disease.

This section begins with a brief overview of research on culturally distinctive ways of coping with illness and maintaining health. Una Maclean argues that we are currently witnessing a renaissance in folk medicine and everyday health promotion and that there has been some increase in anthropological research into health cultures in Europe. This author refers to the influence of ethnicity on health-related behaviour, and social position is considered more generally by Janine Pierret in her exploratory research looking at differences between employment groups in France regarding their views of health and sickness. These views, or interpretations, are presented as reflections of the ways in which people relate to the established social order—in particular, the author argues that the type of work that people do (manual/mental; public/private sector) affects their notions of health and illness, its predictability and preventability. These frameworks for explaining health and illness are shown to have significant implications for reported health behaviour and use of preventive services.

Horst Noack draws upon an overview of a wide range of studies to develop a discussion of relationships between social structure, health, and health behaviour. There are many problems in the conceptualization and measurement of all three key terms, reflecting the current inadequacy of theory. However, data from several countries show a consistently inverse relationship between social position or class and measures of both health and illness. Although there are diverse explanations for this, Noack argues that the poorer health of lower classes is in part a consequence of unfavourable health-related behaviours. The final contribution from Hungary draws upon an insightful analysis of historical influences on behavioural change in that country. The 'risk' factors associated with the deterioration in health status are described in the context of the life cycle and of social, economic, and cultural trends. These have culminated in mortality rates in Hungary that are amongst the highest in Europe. The authors point to negative effects on health behaviour of a rapid socio-economic transition indicating how changes in the family, public policy and the economy may contradict health interests and act as major sources of stress. Their conclusions draw together many of the implications from other papers in this section about the need to co-ordinate multiple strategies—legislation, price policy, town planning, environmental protection, community oraganization—to respond to the diverse influences on health. They show that research which seeks to understand health behaviour must consider individual and societal factors, and their interaction.

4

Ethnographic approaches to health

UNA MACLEAN

A well-established method of learning about people's behaviour in relation to health and illness is that of medical anthropology and there is now an extensive literature on the subject from all over the world. Essentially it depends on lengthy interviews and prolonged detailed note-taking over a period of time by trained observers, who themselves participate as much as possible in the day-to-day lives of their subjects.

Every culture has developed its own distinctive ways and rituals for dealing with sickness, disability, and the danger of death. These approaches are founded upon prevailing beliefs about the nature of the universe and of the relationships within it of individuals to one another, to the gods and to spirits. As well as religious healing activities, which derive from what are regarded as supernatural influences upon health, there are also customary practices of a much more mundane and pragmatic kind, relating to diet, sexual mores, the proper precautions to be taken by pregnant and labouring women, and the details of child care. Appropriate herbal and other medications for a wide range of symptoms and physical conditions are generally to be found, as well as particular individuals, who are locally respected on account of their specialized knowledge about disease causation and treatment regimes.

The subject is complex and eminently worthy of research. It is sometimes called ethnomedicine, itself a branch of ethnoscience. The set of beliefs which prevail in any one place will not be based upon the premises familiar to Western scientists, but they do have an internal consistency of their own and make good sense to those who utilize and practise them. Kleinman (1980) has stressed the different explanatory models which people use in the effort to understand their misfortunes.

In many parts of the world, medicine is not conceived in circumscribed, technical terms, but involves a vast range of accepted and customary ways of avoiding or combating all of life's threats and dangers. The notion of prophylaxis, in the sense of precautionary measures to escape ill health or prevent bad luck, is central to many medical systems throughout the Third World. Even if any particular set of ritual precautions, prescriptions, or protective charms may seem far removed from modern notions of health promotion, on close inspection they may all be seen to fall into the same category of attempts to maximize personal, social, and family welfare. A useful compendium of African therapeutic systems provides many examples of this kind (Ademuwagun *et al*. 1979).

Lately the term 'health culture' has been coined to cover this broad area of human activity and study. It was previously seen as the special preserve of medical anthropologists but folklorists, sometimes regarded as rather less academic, have also contributed to our knowledge and understanding. Recently the World Health Organization has taken note of this important field of research, recognizing that local beliefs and practices must be seriously studied when attempting to introduce the elements of primary health care to any community. Publications have, for instance, appeared on 'traditional practices affecting the health of women and children', drawing attention to the continuance of female circumcision in parts of Africa (WHO 1979). The activities of traditional birth attendants have been extensively documented, as part of the movement to encourage their upgrading (WHO 1985).

Other publications pay tribute to the central role of women in the maintenance of family health (Rutabanzibwa-Ngaiza, J. *et al*. 1985). In 1978, as part of the Declaration of Alma Ata, WHO declared that primary health care would need to involve all kinds of health workers, and should include traditional practitioners, suitably trained, socially and technically, to work as members of a health team and to respond to the expressed needs of their communities. Leaving aside the question of how far these initiatives have so far been reflected in changes in health policy in the countries concerned, what is significant here is the belated realization that we need to recognize the cultural component in health-related behaviour and acknowledge that, throughout much of the Third World, it is usually only traditional practitioners who are available to help the local people (Bannerman *et al*. 1983). The great shortage of other personnel and the world-wide tendency of health professionals to remain in the big towns deprives rural populations of scarce skills and resources.

It would be a grave error to imagine that this is a matter which concerns only those who live and work in the Third World. Scientific or modern medicine rests upon premises which are still poorly understood or accepted by many potential patients and a whole range of other systems of explanation and therapy can be found to co-exist, in both America and Europe. Just as there is now a move to treat traditional, African and Indian, medicine more seriously so we have become aware of the extent and variety of forms of 'alternative' medicine, each with their own notions of disease causation and health enhancement. Homeopathy, chiropractice, naturo-therapy, and faith healing are only a few examples. In addition, acupuncture and bio-feedback methods are commonly practised, whilst increasing numbers of people today try to maintain and improve their own health by special regimes of diet, exercise and herbal remedies. Folk medicine, far from disappearing, is manifesting a renaissance.

Apart from the specific matter of using or trusting alternative medicine, people vary widely in their immediate and customary responses to symptoms. Ethnicity is one significant factor here, as was demonstrated some time ago in America by Zborowski (1952) and Zola (1966). The influence of race on health-related behaviour is also clearly apparent in Britain among immigrants who have come from the Indian subcontinent and the West Indies. Transcultural psychiatrists were among the first to document the striking contrasts in the way patients presented, according to whether or not they belonged to an Anglo-Saxon background, but there are now a rapidly expanding number of articles on race and health (Johnson 1983).

Even among people of the same race, notable differences can exist regarding what are considered as departures from customary health and about whether or when professional help is needed. A proper appreciation of these matters demands an ethnographic approach. It is not sufficient to subject samples of populations to a set of predetermined questions, using classical social survey techniques, since it is inevitable that the unexpected explanations and accounts held by respondents will be precisely those which are liable to escape the imagination of the survey designer. But, whereas anthropological approaches, involving in-depth interviews and participant observation, have now become commonplace in developing countries, their use in Europe has hitherto been somewhat exceptional. No doubt the reasons for this deficit must partly lie in the policies of research-funding bodies. Several examples, however, are worthy of mention. Tuula Vaskilampi has pioneered the study of surviving folk medicine practices in Finland (Vaskilampi and MacCormack 1982). Claudine Herzlich (1973) has helped us realize how middle-class urban Frenchwomen envisage illness. Vieda Skultans (1974) has provided a picture of the support which unhappy Welsh women derive from spiritualism. Cecil Helman (1984) has uncovered traces of old, humoral notions of sickness causation among well-to-do Surrey suburbanites. Mildred Blaxter, in the course of studying two generations of poor women in Aberdeen, has revealed the stoicism with which grandmothers faced previous severe difficulties and disease in their families (Blaxter and Patterson 1982). Sarah Cunningham-Burley has been casting light on the way contemporary young mothers monitor their infants' behaviour for the first signs of ill health (Cunningham-Burley and Maclean 1985).

If we are in the business of health promotion in the widest sense we should always remain sensitive to the enormous number of ways of defining health and disease which are held by ordinary people. Certainly we cannot teach others about health without appreciating their own current beliefs. Perhaps we can also learn from them. The ethnographic approach should not be reserved for exotic, foreign cultures. It is needed close at hand.

References

Ademuwagun, Z. A., Ayoade, J. A., Hanson, I. E., and Warren, D. M. (eds) (1979). *African therapeutic systems*. Crossroads Press, Brandeis University.

Bannerman, H., Burton, J., and Ch'en Wen-Chieh (eds) (1983). *Traditional medicine and health care coverage*. World Health Organization, Geneva.

Blaxter, M. and Patterson, E. (1982). *Mothers and daughters: a three generational study of health attitudes and behaviour*. Heinemann Educational Books, London.

Cunningham-Burley, S. and Maclean, U. (1985). *Expectations and evidence: the cultural context of childhood illness*. Mimeographed Report, Edinburgh University.

Helman, C. (1984). *Culture, health and illness: an introduction for health professionals*. Wright, Bristol.

Herzlich, C. (1973). *Health and illness*. Academic Press, London.

Johnson, M. R. D. (1983). *Race and health*. A select bibliography, S.S.R.C. Centre for Research in Ethnic Relations, University of Warwick, Coventry.

Kleinman, A. (1980). *Patients and healers in the context of culture*. University of California Press, Berkeley.

Rutabanzibwa-Ngaiza, J., Heggenhougan, K. and Watt, G. (1985). *Women and health in Africa*. Evaluation and Planning Centre for Health Care, London School of Hygiene and Tropical Medicine.

Skultans, V. (1974). *Intimacy and ritual*. Routledge and Kegan Paul, London.

Vaskilampi, T. and MacCormack, C. P. (eds) (1982). *Folk medicine and health culture: the role of folk medicine in modern health care*. Kuopio, Finland.

WHO (1979). *Traditional practices affecting the health of women and children*. Report of a seminar in Khartoum, WHO Regional Office for the Eastern Mediterranean, Alexandria.

WHO (1985). *Traditional birth attendants: a resource for the health of women*. Joint WHO/FIGO Task Force for the promotion of maternal and child health. Elsevier, Amsterdam.

Zborowski, M. (1952). Cultural components in response to pain. *Journal of Social Issues* **8**, 16–30.

Zola, I. K. (1966). Culture and symptoms: an analysis of patients' presenting complaints. *American Sociological Review* **31**, 615–30.

5

What social groups think they can do about health

JANINE PIERRET

Abstract

Even though, nowadays in our society, the domain of illness undeniably appertains to the medical system, the complete survey of this domain in all its complexity cannot be made with reference to this institutional system alone. For more than 20 years now, sociologists have tried to show that illness is as much a social as an objective, natural, or physical phenomenon. Interpretations of health and illness express the ways in which individuals and groups are related to the established social order. In this sense, they are special means for expressing the relations between body, nature, and society.

The aim here is to use the qualitative results of an in-depth analysis of 130 non-directive interviews about health and illness in order to bring to light the global frameworks of interpretation wherein can be seen the complex relationships between these two notions (health, illness) and work, risk, uncertainty, and prevention. It is argued that the position that an individual has within the system of production affects his way of thinking about and of interpreting his relations with society. What interviewees said that they do for their health cannot be understood without referring to their conceptual, or representational, frameworks wherein health and illness are used to bridge the gap between the biological and social spheres.

Meanings of health

In everyday conversation, few topics come up as often as health and illness. People discuss, interpret, and judge these preoccupying topics in terms that go beyond 'medicine' or the 'body'. Even though, nowadays in our society, the domain of illness undeniably appertains to the medical system, the complete survey of this domain in all its complexity cannot be made with reference to this institutional system alone. For more than 20 years now, the social sciences have attempted to show that illness is as much a social as an objective, natural, or physical phenomenon. Interpretations of health and illness express the ways in which individuals and groups are related to the established social order. In this sense, they are special means for expressing the relations between body, nature and society. Through the study of these 'collective representations', French sociologists have tried to show that conceptions of health and illness have their own coherency, independently of the categories of medical terminology. Thanks to this research, it can be seen that these conceptions provide a means of observing a society's values and beliefs.

The conclusions drawn from these studies, even though they may not directly answer the questions that the medical profession ask about people's behaviour towards health, should nevertheless enable health professionals both to place their actions in a broader perspective and to enquire into the effectiveness of their policies. For instance, the *Comité Français d'Education pour la Santé* realized that providing information and education do not by themselves make people change their life styles and do 'what's good for their health'. Although health tends to be a central value in our society, it does not have the same meaning to everyone.

Concepts of health among workers in France

The results presented here are drawn from the second phase of a research project begun in 1979. With stratification by age, sex, and socio-economic status, 130 persons were selected in a quarter of Paris, the department of Essone, and southern France. Non-directive interviews of an hour and a half were carried out with each person who was asked, 'I would like you to talk to me about health, about what it means to you.' These taped interviews, once transcribed, were analysed comparatively in order to bring to light the shared 'discourses' held in common by most of them. This reconstructing of discourses revealed four different frameworks of interpretation. These frameworks, which individuals develop in order to give meaning to their diverse practices, shed light on the complex relations between health, work, risk, uncertainty, and prevention (Pierret 1984).

This second phase of research has used the aforementioned material in order to define groups which are homogeneous with respect to members' jobs. Five groups were constructed by combining several variables: qualifications, level of education, the job actually held, the sector (whether private or public) wherein it is located, and the degree of involvement in the production process. This accounted for 65 interviewees: 33 men and 32 women; 31 over 40 years old; 25 dwelling in Paris, 23 in Essone and 17 in southern France. The following hypothesis underlies this research: the type of work that people do affects the way that they interpret notions of health and illness.

The first two groups—farmers and those workers directly participating as they do in production—use their bodies as tools or implements. Their conceptions of risk and illness, though differing, do have in common the idea of unpredictability. The three other groups, which belong to the 'middle classes', own what we might call cultural capital: their jobs in the tertiary sector require know-how and training. The type of employment, whether private or public, strongly affects their views of the world.

Let me emphasize before going on to discuss each of these groups that the following comments have come out of what people said they do and not out of observations of what they actually do. There is no simple relationship between behaviour and the framework of interpretation that members of a social group have constructed in order both to give a meaning to their practices and to define their place within society. Any explanation of actual behaviour would have to take into account these frameworks along with other factors (for instance, the person's objective situation and the supply of health care).

The *small farmers* in our survey made coherent, homogeneous comments about the relationship between work, health, and nature. The cycle of the seasons imposes a rhythm and organization upon both work and household activities (meals, sleep, etc.). Sickness befalls as unpredictably as drought or frost. Like plants or animals, people are menaced by illness and death.

Good health is good fortune. Farmers declared that sound health is the most valuable possession. It is the mainstay of their lives. Thanks to it, they can work. Without it, nothing is possible. This conception of health as a value, as wealth, has come from a distant past, from the rural economy and a society that toils. Health is, to an extent, a capital that a farmer owns from birth, a capital that he can bestow upon his children. Indispensable to his work, good health is sustained and developed by the 'healthfulness' of this work, which increases resistance against disease. In the farm world, work governs and organizes people's lives, and farmers continually have to face up to this fact. Consequently, interviewees said that they do not have time to tend or pay attention to themselves. They are too busy to fall sick.

These small farmers considered illness to be a natural, usually unforesee-able event associated with the weather, animals, and water. However, it does not stop them from going about their activities, somehow they adjust to it. Work prevails over all else; it cannot wait. Colds, influenza, or fevers do not keep a farmer from working, and he does not go to a doctor's surgery before being seriously ill. When he falls sick, his family is the first to take care of him. For family members, sickness is part of living; and living implies ageing, this wear and tear of passing time, and dying.

Farmers associated the idea of foreseeing with that of forestalling, predict-ing with preventing. The very idea of prevention is a threat because it brings illness into one's midst whenever there is no cause for alarm. Prevention means warning people in order to scare them or make them worry. None the less respondents did not forget to mention precautions taken in their work (for instance, vaccinations against tetanus, veterinary controls or safety devices on tractors). However, such measures affect not their health but their principle preoccupation, work. In short, nothing can be done for health; it is an essential attribute: a person either is well or is not. He can fight against sickness only when it attacks.

Sickness worries farmers inasmuch as it makes their existence precarious. It is a natural contingency, a chance happening that must be faced in a world of toil that is subject both to nature's rhythm and to the constraints imposed by the industrialization of the market in their sector.

Unskilled or semi-skilled workers holding insecure jobs, the second group in this survey, mainly worried over material difficulties. For them, sound health opens the way to employment and thus to acceptance and integration since only a job proves a person's worth and ensures his place within society. Sickness, because it upsets a fragile balance, was considered to be a handicap that keeps one from fulfilling one's obligations at work and at home. It symbolizes the worker's vulnerability to the contingencies of everyday life.

For these workers, sickness is a constant menace that unforseeably fells people. It has many causes, among them: working conditions, food, climate, weather, germs, heredity, or contagion. Respondents distinguished clearly between what they considered to be normal, mild, or commonplace illnesses (for instance, infectious as well as childhood diseases) and serious conditions (resulting from pulmonary or cardiovascular diseases, cancer, or accidents). When questioned, they placed illnesses in a temporal perspective. Accordingly, an ordinary disease can lead to complications or chronic states that compel the sick person to withdraw from the labour force.

Whereas health is a vital force to one's life project, sickness, along with worsened living or working conditions (in particular, pollution, alcohol, tobacco, and artificial products in food) wear the body down and out. These are the factors which inverviewees had in mind when they said that they are careful whenever they can be. They talked much about working conditions (the reduced workforce, speeded-up assembly lines, new production quotas, heat and noise at the workplace, etc.), but they thought that job-related risks to their health can hardly be lessened, not even through the action of labour unions. They do try to control their consumption of food, tobacco, and alcohol and their participation in physical activities. In doing this, however, they meet up with material and financial limitations. For example, those who would like to eat fresh, natural food admitted that such foods tend to be much more expensive and beyond their means. Interviewees weighed the consequences of addiction to alcohol or tobacco, and argued for the need to take appropriate steps, for instance, to stop smoking if 'there's something wrong with the lungs'. Apparently out of a belief that 'the sooner, the better', they voiced the hope that the campaign against smoking will, through the schools, influence young people who have not yet taken up the habit.

In spite of suggesting ways to resist the unrelating forces that wear the body out, these workers thought that such precautions are not very effective. Since sickness is a constant threat, what counts is to have the means to be able to react as need be; in particular, to have access to health-care services and facilities. This social group wants better, regular in-depth check-ups at the workplace and free health care. A symbol of the vulnerability of these workers who hold insecure jobs; sickness is unpredictable and implies being able, whenever it attacks, to react, especially through guaranteed access to health care.

The third group included executive secretaries, draughtsmen, industrial photographers, and other technicians employed by private firms. For these *vocationally-trained, mid-level, white-collar workers in the private sector*, health is, above all, an objective to be reached, or even a life-goal understood in individualistic, hedonistic terms. Illness is, therefore, a hindrance to the individual's pursuit of happiness. People should be capable of weighing the consequences of acts so as to draw the right conclusions and 'manage' their lives more efficiently. These white-collar workers act for the sake of their health, actions that reflect their feelings about the 'duty to be healthy'. Their framework of interpretation seeks to resolve the contradictions between the pursuit of happiness by an individual and the limitations set by society.

These attempts by white-collar personnel to 'manage their lives' can be seen in their choice of practices normally associated with pleasure, namely smoking, eating, and drinking. Interviewees emphasized the pleasure of having a healthy, balanced diet and of gathering with one's family or friends around a table. The consumption of alcohol and tobacco, which concerns them squarely, is a topic about which they voiced firm opinions. Accordingly, drinking and smoking are consequences of the ever-increasing difficulties and annoyances of modern life; they are a way to relax, 'unwind' and indulge in a little fun. The harmful effects of the misuse of alcohol or tobacco are placed within the larger setting of a society which exposes everyone to risks (pollution, working conditions, the hurried pace of life, etc.). Members of this social group object to advertising campaigns which make people feel guilty about smoking, drinking, or eating certain foodstuffs. They claim the 'right to be crazy, to have fun' and refuse an aseptic society of well-balanced people all behaving reasonably. For them, tobacco and alcohol are signs of a society which no longer knows how to take time to live and which produces sickness. Nevertheless each individual must weigh the risks and make his own decisions.

Emphasizing as they did that people are free to choose, these private sector white-collar workers did not seem very worried about sickness. In addition to the troubles of modern living (stress, worry, and so forth), they mainly mentioned ordinary infectious diseases which are not very serious. Apparently, the major effect of illness is to keep them from exercising their free will.

The fourth group, to which we refer as *mid-level, white-collar workers in the public sector*, was made up of primary school teachers and employees in public administrations. Members of this group had not pursued education beyond secondary school. Their approach to health issues is collective and institutional. Interviewees usually talked about the need of a different health policy rather than about personal efforts (which they considered to be not very effective) or about their private health worries.

For these white-collar workers, sickness has many causes: working and housing conditions, the pace of life, pollution, isolation in big cities, and the excessive consumption of food, tobacco, or alcohol. Illness reflects and reinforces social inequality. Respondents did not talk much about personal practices (for instance, smoking, eating, or drinking), but they did point out the value of physical exercise. In their opinion, only the community or its institutions can act upon health and lead people, especially through education, to adopt other habits. For example, schools and companies could offer first-aid courses or encourage contributions to blood banks; and cafeterias at school or at work could help spread knowledge about nutrition.

None the less the ultimate solutions are to be sought within the system of medical institutions. According to these white-collar workers, a different health policy would help reduce inequality. New health-care facilities should be set up, and their services provided free. The larger number of facilities would make it possible to treat the ill and illness differently. Interviewees were in favour of developing 'social medicine' (through dispensaries, maternal and child-care services, etc.). They also suggested new kinds of neighbourhood services: grouping physicians' surgeries or establishing health centres that would, for instance, organize educative meetings for health-care users. Furthermore, they advocated the development and improvement of preventive medicine, notably at the workplace and in schools.

For public sector white-collar workers, sickness results from and reinforces social inequality. Reducing this inequality calls for collective, institutional measures which the medical system can apply, whence the need for a different health policy that should be founded both upon the provision of medical care free of charge in order to improve the access to health-care services and upon 'social medicine' in order to develop a view of public health issues. These measures should be completed by others having to do with preventive medicine.

For *college-educated secondary school teachers*, the fifth group in this survey, illness is a social problem caused by modern society. By society, this notion round which their comments turn, they mean consumer society, industrial society, city life, and the system of political power as well. These teachers are seemingly torn between recognizing the worth of scientific progress and criticizing its effects, especially upon the pace and quality of everyday life. Although they tend to be in favour of progress, they weigh the pros and cons but refuse to consider the idea of having to pay the price. Compared with members of the other groups, they insisted more upon social measures, political actions, and government interventions for, otherwise, individuals' efforts would be ineffective.

Those secondary school teachers condemned the urban way of life that breeds illness, menaces a person's equilibrium and causes more and more behavioural disorders and mental illnesses. What they described forms a whole, coherent system that comprises all sorts of conditions—working, commuting, housing, environmental—all of which act upon each other so as to upset the equilibrium necessary to well-being. Illness is produced by society, it is part of society, it necessitates both remedial and preventive measures. Although they pointed to the curative powers of medicine as a symbol of society's technical and scientific progress, these teachers criticized the medical profession for the way that it uses its know-how. In favour of the qualitative and quantitative development of the medical infrastructure, interviewees, even though they agreed on the necessity of medical interventions, did not think that these would suffice for reducing the causes of illness. Medicine can only remedy what society has bred as a result of inequality. Given the conditions underlying this inequality, health problems have much less to do with medicine than with political actions in favour of social justice.

The notion of prevention, which lies at the centre of teachers' conceptions of collective health care, enables them to reconcile their view of society with their belief in progress. They emphasized preventive medicine, which has proven its efficacy by applying new discoveries and techniques. However, since the roots of sickness run deeply throughout society, check-ups and vaccinations do not suffice. A system has to be set up for treating the social aetiology of illness, a system that would, in other words, 'go to the roots' and treat the actual conditions of illness (pollution, working conditions, and so forth). In line with the belief in progress, prevention implies understanding the social determinants of sickness. By adopting this position, these teachers were able to reconcile their favourable opinion about the application of scientific and technical knowledge with their demands for interventions in the social sphere.

For secondary school teachers, illness, because it is caused by modern society, necessitates collective measures which should be centred around prevention. Since they believe that society should profit from advances in science and technology, these teachers favour developing a policy of prevention that goes beyond the medical field and reaches down to the 'roots' of the problem. To delve so deeply, this policy must combine knowledge about how society is organized with knowledge about medicine.

Conclusion

The position that an individual has within the system of production affects his way of thinking about and of interpreting his relations with society. What interviewees said that they do for their health cannot be understood without referring to their conceptual, or representational, frameworks wherein health and illness are used to bridge the gap between the biological and social spheres, to treat—or might I not say 'cure'—the relations between themselves and society.

Reference

Pierret, J. (1984). Significations sociales de la santé: Paris, l'Essone, l'Hérault. In *Le Sens du mal: anthropologie, histoire, sociologie de la maladie* (ed. M. Augé and C. Herzlich), pp. 217–46. Editions des Archives Contemporaines, Paris.

6

The role of socio-structural factors in health behaviour

HORST NOACK

'Over 99% of us are born healthy and made sick as a result of personal misbehaviour and environmental conditions.' (Knowles 1977, p. 58)

'The essence of the second revolution in public health is the recognition that the central issues to be addressed involve the modification of the social environments.' (Maddox 1985, p. 30)

The problem

This chapter addresses a question which is of considerable practical and scientific relevance: What social factors are associated with health-related behaviours and how do they influence such behaviours?

In dealing with this question we face three difficulties. First, both the concept of social structure and the concept of health behaviour are not at all simple and carry a variety of meanings. Secondly, health-related behaviours are, by definition, linked to another broad concept, the notion of health. Thirdly, both health behaviour and health are socially defined and influenced by social structure.

For these reasons we found it difficult to address the role of socio-structural factors in health behaviour in a straightforward manner. Rather, we selected a conceptual framework (Fig. 6.1) which we believe helps to sort out the difficulties inherent in our question and to deal with them more easily.

According to the links between the three key terms, the chapter is divided into three parts. In the second section we review some of the literature on the relationships between social conditions and dimensions of health. The third section summarizes research results on the association between health-related behaviours and health. In the fourth section we deal with the links between aspects of social structure and health-related behaviours. Drawing upon more recent social theory, we attempt to integrate in a final section the major findings summarized in this chapter into a general theoretical framework of social structure and health-related action. Furthermore, we suggest scientific research and evaluation studies which eventually may throw light

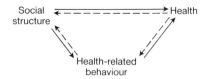

Fig. 6.1 Conceptual framework of health-related behaviour.

on the social factors and social processes that help to stabilize or change health-related behaviours and hence health.

Social conditions of ill-health and health

It is well known that premature death, ill-health and health are unequally distributed in society. Many epidemiological investigations were undertaken to study similarities and differences among socio-economic and socio-cultural groups in mortality, morbidity, and also positive health.

Social class

Mortality rates are still the best available indicators of health or rather ill-health. In Europe, North America, and Australia mortality rates were consistently found to be inversely related to occupational class, socio-economic group, level of education and income. Social class differences were observed for nearly all disease categories and for males and females at all ages (Antonovsky 1967; Klein 1980; Townsend and Davidson 1982; Hunt *et al*. 1985).

Most available indicators of morbidity reveal a similar picture. For example, in Britain, work days lost because of illness or injury are strongly and inversely associated with occupational class, and rates of self-reported limiting, long-standing illness were considerably higher among unskilled workers than among skilled workers and professionals (Townsend and Davidson 1982). Coronary heart disease and risk factors of cardiovascular disease, in particular elevated blood pressure, were found more frequently among the lower socio-economic groups (Rose and Marmot 1981; Theorell *et al*. 1984). Not only somatic disease but also mental illness and psychiatric symptoms tended to be more prevalent among the lower social classes (Goldberg and Huxley 1980).

Some research results on positive health complement this picture. Thus, level of self-reported well-being, fulfilment, fitness, independence, and social functioning, as well as absence of physical and psychological problems, were found to be positively related to indicators of social class (Blaxter 1985;

Buchmann *et al*. 1985; Hunt *et al*. 1985; Marmot and Morris 1984; Slater *et al*. 1985).

Several alternative explanations were advanced to account for the social class differences in health: natural and social selection, socio-structural factors and cultural factors (Townsend and Davidson 1982). The structuralist ('materialist') explanation sees the reason for the higher rates of ill-health among the lower social classes as being due to their relatively deprived, more hazardous and more strenuous conditions of living and work. According to the cultural explanation the main reason is assumed to be the specific life-style of the lower classes which is characterized by a relatively high prevalence of so-called risk behaviours. In discussing the results of one of the most impressive studies of the impact of social and behavioural factors on health, the Alameda County study, Berkman and Syme (1979) conclude that the striking difference in mortality between the highest and the lowest educational classes cannot be explained by specific social and behavioural variables. These and other authors (Cassel 1974; Henry and Stephens 1977; Antonovsky and Shoham 1978) suggest that we should investigate how social conditions affect general susceptibility, resistance resources and coping behaviour.

Culture

A number of studies have shown cultural factors to play a significant role in the development of Western diseases (e.g. Henry and Stephens 1977).

Studies of acculturation have provided particularly valuable insights into the importance of social conditions and health-related practices. For example, the incidence rates of gastrointestinal cancers among Japanese immigrants in Hawaii differ from the incidence rates in Japan and are quite similar to the rates of the white Hawaiian population (Doll and Peto 1981). The prevalence of coronary heart disease of Japanese-Americans in California who retained their traditional culture has remained at the low level found in Japan, whereas in those who assimilated the American culture it has risen to levels close to the American rates (Marmot and Syme, 1976).

Striking differences in the rates of modern diseases were also observed within countries. Thus, the rate of coronary heart disease in an American town with a Catholic population of Italian descent was only half the rate of a Protestant population of German/English descent living in a similar town. The Catholic-Italian culture was characterized as the more 'easy' one, in terms of social cohesiveness, social disruption, and low level of tension: there was no apparent difference in nutrition (Henry and Stephens 1977).

Social networks

At least since Durkheim's (1897) well-known work on suicide, social ties as well as social solidarity and support have been assumed to affect health.

More recent research suggests that these factors play a key role in the development of disease and the maintenance and improvement of health. Thus, mortality rates as well as rates of chronic somatic illness and of psychiatric disturbance tend to be lower among the married than among the unmarried, separated, or divorced (Goldberg and Huxley 1980; Fox and Goldblatt 1982).

In the Alameda County study already referred to, those participants with extensive social networks were less likely to die in the nine years of follow-up than people with little or no social support. This association was independent of self-reported health practices, socio-economic group, and health status at the beginning of the study. Similarly, the social network had a significant independent effect on future self-reported health status (Berkman and Breslow 1983).

A distinct contribution of social support to health was demonstrated in several other studies. For example, under stressful social conditions lack of support was clearly associated with clinical depression in women (Brown and Harris 1978) and perceived symptoms of distress (Dressler 1985a).

Integration into a supportive social network and a high sense of control over one's life situation was found to be correlated with perceived positive health (Seeman *et al*. 1985). These and several other research results corroborate the notion of social support as representing an effective buffer against psychosocial strains in social and occupational roles (LaRocco *et al*. 1980; Thoits 1982). From a specific sociological perspective (Giddens 1979) the social network can be viewed as a system of interdependent social action which affects ill-health and health.

Work

Although work has long been suspected of playing a crucial role in the distribution of health and disease, there exists a great dearth of research in this field. Whereas physical and chemical occupational hazards have been studied more extensively, research into the social condition and psychosocial processes of work is relatively recent. For example, in one of the larger field studies, self-reported symptoms and diseases as well as medically diagnosed hypertension were found to be related to perceived occupational stress of factory workers (House *et al*. 1979). In occupations with high levels of psycho-social job strain the prevalence of coronary heart disease was significantly higher than in low-strain occupations (Karasek *et al*. 1982a; Theorell *et al*. 1984).

Social factors which are related to job strain were shown to be excessive psychological demands, such as a hectic pace of work and at the same time limited decision latitude and little intellectual stimulation (Karasek *et al*. 1982b). On the other hand, work which is perceived as meaningful and wherein people get involved may represent an important coping resource (Benner 1984).

Gender

Across the social classes marked gaps in ill-health and health have been observed between men and women. In Britain for example, where mortality rates have approximately halved over the last 100 years, mortality rates for men have remained substantially higher than for women. In fact the mortality rate for men has increased relative to that for women over the last decades (McKeown 1976). However, despite lower mortality women tend to report more physical symptoms than men (Waldron 1983), more limiting chronic illness and more days of restricted activity (OPCS 1984). Similarly, most studies show higher rates of psychosomatic and psychoneurotic conditions for women than for men (Goldberg and Huxley 1980).

Although the complex factors or mechanisms underlying these differences (including the genetic ones) are far from being understood (Waldron 1983), the available evidence seems to suggest that women tend to experience more role-specific psychosocial strains than men, perceive health problems somewhat differently from men, and engage in different kinds of health behaviour (Kandel *et al.* 1985; Gove 1984; Verbrugge 1985).

In summary, there is some indication that the marked gaps in mortality, morbidity, and positive health observed between social classes or socio-economic group may be explained, at least in part, by three aspects of social structure: social position and the demands of private and occupational social roles; the social network and related patterns of instrumental and socio-emotional support; and the specific lifestyle patterns, behavioural orientations, beliefs, and knowledge summarized under the notion of culture. From this point of view, health-related behaviour can be considered an important link between socio-structural factors and health, as well as an inherent aspect of social structure.

Health-related behaviours and health

Before dealing with the links between social structure and health-related behaviour we will consider the potential impacts of such behaviour on health. In terms of both theoretical and empirical work this seems to be a rather neglected scientific field. With the exception of Antonovsky's (1981) salutogenic model, hardly any theoretical framework exists. This lack of theory appears to be one of the reasons for the difficulties in defining and analysing health-related behaviour in a wider socio-economic, cultural, and psychosocial context.

From a sociological and socio-psychological perspective three broad categories of health-related behaviour might be distinguished:

- *Health-promoting behaviour*. This category comprises various kinds of social action which, from the actor's point of view, are intentionally directed towards the maintenance or improvement of health and the prevention of disease—in Weberian terms, instrumental or goal-directed actions.
- *Health-related practices*. These are regular routine practices which form an integral part of everyday life. As standardized modes of behaviour these practices tend to be specific to institutions such as the primary social or kinship group and to the occupation. Although not intentionally directed towards specific health goals they do have an impact on health.
- *Coping behaviours*. These are behaviours which people tend to produce in order to reduce psychological distress or to protect themselves against real or expected harmful psychological and physical experiences. Coping behaviours may be unintended or automatic reactions or they may be goal-directed and planned actions.

While these categories refer to actions or activities which frequently are viewed as individual behaviours they may, in fact, represent social behaviours or collective health behaviour (Green 1984).

Health-promoting behaviours

Although there will be little dissent that some goal-directed behaviours (for example, giving up smoking) are likely to improve health and protect against disease, the value of others may be disputed (for example, switching to a particular diet). Only limited research seems to have been undertaken in this field, for example as part of the Alameda County study. In this study the group of adults who reported using preventive medical services showed a slightly lower mortality rate during the nine year follow-up than those who had not reported this behaviour. This effect was independent of high-risk health practices such as smoking, overeating, or having very little or too much sleep (Berkman and Syme 1979; Berkman and Breslow 1983).

Health-related practices

The most convincing evidence about the impact of regular health-related practices on future health was also provided by the Alameda County study (Berkman and Breslow 1983). For both men and women and for all age groups included, five so-called high-risk practices were found to be strongly, and each one independently, associated with mortality during the follow-up period of nine years. These risk practices were smoking cigarettes, consuming excessive quantities of alcohol, being physically inactive, being obese or underweight and sleeping fewer than seven or more than eight hours per night. In a separate analysis, a similar relationship was found for two additional health practices: skipping breakfast and 'snacking' instead of eating regular meals.

A health practice index defined as the number of high-risk practices predicted total mortality as well as mortality from coronary heart disease, other cardiovascular disease and cancer, independently of socio-economic status, social support, race and several psychological factors. Furthermore, these high-risk practices predicted an index of health status over time, each one independently and more strongly when additively combined into an index. Again, this relationship was independent of social support, income and education. Thus, each of the socio-economic variables, the network index and the health-practices index was shown to make a significant independent contribution to future health (Berkman and Breslow 1983).

This conclusion was supported by a number of other studies. For example, epidemiological and clinical research indicated that physical activity can delay, if not prevent, the onset and reduce the severity of several of the major chronic degenerative diseases (Haskell 1985). Perceived positive health was found to be influenced by individual health habits, independently of socio-economic group (Slater *et al*. 1985). A cognitive element of health-related practices, general positive health orientation, together with sufficient social support, was shown to be associated with 'stamina in later life' (Colerick 1985).

Coping behaviours

In this field, most research has focused on what is being interpreted as a particular form of risky coping behaviour, the so-called coronary-prone or Type A behaviour pattern. In a prospective study of middle-aged Californian men, Type A participants were found to have higher rates of coronary heart disease and myocardial infarction than Type B participants (Rosenman *et al*. 1975). While similar findings were obtained in the Framingham heart study (Haynes and Feinleib 1982), other studies failed to show any relationship.

A cohort study of West German workers seems to suggest an interactive effect of situational factors and coping behaviour. Only in the group of workers exposed to high job-strain was a particular vigorous coping style associated with elevated levels of blood pressure and LDL cholesterol, in the low-job-strain group no such association was found (Siegrist 1984). Several authors (e.g. Buchmann *et al*. 1985; Marmot and Morris 1984; Matarazzo 1984) interpret high-risk practices such as smoking, overeating and excessive alcohol consumption, as effective coping behaviours in situations experienced as psychologically distressing.

Little evidence, however, is available on the presumed positive health impacts of coping. As suggested by an Israeli study (Ben-Sira 1985) feelings of confidence in one's own competence (potency) and a perception of society as being meaningful and predictable tend to have a buffering effect against social tensions and increase health balance. In a study conducted in a black American community a particularly active coping style had positive effects on stress reduction in women but not in men (Dressler 1985b), thus pointing towards coping as an interactive process.

From this brief review of some of the literature on the links between health-related behaviours and health two conclusions can be drawn: First, health-related practices tend to have a strong and independent effect on mortality as well as on future ill-health and health. Secondly, although there is some indication of positive effects, so far too little research has been undertaken to draw any firm conclusion about the contribution of health-promoting and coping behaviours on health.

As we have shown, health-related behaviours represent a very wide spectrum of person–environment interactions or transactions. In order to analyse and categorize them it is important to take into account the social context, the interaction of the actor or the group of actors, his/her or their health motivations, the time dimension and the meaning of such behaviours from the individual actor's or the group's point of view. Only to the extent this is done can the influence of socio-structural factors in health behaviour be understood.

Health-related behaviours and social structure

Before discussing the intricate inter-relationship between social structure and health-related behaviours in a more systematic way, we will review some of the related empirical research.

Health-promoting behaviours

A relatively large number of studies on preventive health behaviour were conducted, most of them in the tradition of the health belief model (Rosenstock 1966). Quite consistently it was shown that two psychosocial factors, 'perceived barriers' to health action and 'perceived susceptibility' to a specific disease, are strong predictors of preventive health behaviour, such as using health services for a dental or a physical check-up (Janz and Becker 1984). Unfortunately, little attention has been paid to the question of how these psychosocial determinants of health-promoting behaviour are associated with socio-structural factors.

Research into the social conditions related to preventive health behaviours has been conducted in the United States and in Europe. For example, a British study on women showed a clear relationship between knowledge about the role of diet, smoking and physical exercise in health, on the one hand, and social class on the other. A similar relationship was found between social class and the use of health services for such diverse preventive procedures as dental check-up, cervical smear test, or breast examination. If health services were used for one such examination it was unlikely that they were used for another one (Calnan 1985). In another British study significant class differences were observed between such health-related actions as family planning, antenatal booking, and breast-feeding (Morris 1979).

In a Swiss survey persons with higher education tended to use professional preventive services more frequently than less well-educated persons; and persons in urban areas tended to use them more frequently than persons in rural areas (Buchmann *et al*. 1985).

Health-related practices

Most research in this field investigated how health-related practices are distributed among social classes or socio-economic groups. In Britain the prevalence of so-called risk-behaviours was found to be inversely related to social class (Marmot and Morris 1984). As is known from surveys conducted during the past 20 years, people in the lower occupational classes consistently smoked more cigarettes than people in the middle and upper classes. The diet of the lower classes was relatively high on white bread, sugar, and preserves, and low on wholemeal or brown bread, cheese, fruit, and vitamins. Lower class people reported less leisure-time activity than middle and upper class people.

Similar results were obtained in American studies. The number of positive health practices (according to the list of the Alameda County study) was correlated with level of education, level of occupation, and family income (Slater *et al*. 1985). Also in the United States drinking problems were observed more frequently in the lower social status groups than in the higher ones (Calahan and Cisin 1976). In Switzerland no clear-cut relationship between drinking behaviour and level of education or income was observed (Wüthrich 1979).

Coping behaviours

Relatively little research has so far been conducted into the social distribution of coping behaviours. An American study investigated the effectiveness of several coping styles in marriage, child rearing, household roles, and occupational roles. Coping was found to be most effective in the private and least effective in the occupational roles. Coping resources were observed to be rather unequally distributed in society. Men were able to use more effective coping techniques than women, and better educated and wealthy people used more effective coping than the less well-educated and the poor (Pearlin and Schooler 1978).

As shown by another American study, coping style tends to depend upon the social situation. Thus in work contexts and in situations requiring information more problem-focused coping was found, in health contexts more emotion-focused coping. While in work situations men used more problem-focused coping than women, there was no gender difference in emotion-focused coping (Folkman and Lazarus 1980).

In a study mentioned earlier, occupations were seen to differ in terms of psychosocial and also in physical strain (Karasek *et al*. 1982b). It can thus be expected that occupational groups will tend to differ in their coping behaviours.

The research reviewed in this section suggests marked differences between the social classes or socio-economic groups with regard to their health-promoting behaviours, health-related practices and coping behaviours. In general the lower classes are likely to be less well-protected against health risks and more frequently exposed to situations, activities, and experiences that are detrimental to health. As a number of health-related behaviours, especially regular health-related practices, tend to exert long-term effects on health, it may be concluded that the excess mortality and morbidity of the lower classes, as well as their lower level of overall health are in part a consequence of unfavourable health-related behaviours.

Thus social class does seem to be a highly powerful concept in predicting health and ill-health, even though it is only defined in terms of occupational prestige, level of education or income—that is, in dimensions which clearly oversimplify the social variable (McQueen and Siegrist 1982). However, in order to understand the social factors and processes that make social class such a powerful concept, a far better theoretical grasp is needed than the categories used in sociological, psychological and epidemiological research. One particular problem is that traditional sociological theory lacks a well-advanced theory of action (Giddens 1979). Such a theory would allow us to 'connect' socio-structural variables with health-related behaviours.

What is needed is a theoretical framework suitable for defining social structure, analysing the links between social structure and health-related behaviours, and planning fruitful research. This is of course a formidable task. In the final section we shall limit ourselves to a brief outline of what we consider important elements of such a framework. Using these elements we will try to summarize the findings of the previous sections and to indicate some implications for future research.

On the role of socio-structural factors in health-related behaviours

Implicit in the title of this paper is the plausible assumption, or rather assertion, of a causal relationship between social structure and health-related behaviours. This assertion implies two questions: What are important socio-structural conditions associated with health-related behaviours? What are the processes that govern the continuity of health-related behaviours as well as changes in such behaviours.

To deal with these questions requires a suitable definition of social structure. Following the work of Giddens (1979) on central problems in social theory we find it useful to conceptualize social structure in terms of two properties of the social system, social rules and social resources. By *social system* Giddens refers to the network of reproduced relations between actors or collectivities which express themselves as regularized patterns of social interaction or practice. Relations between actors and collectivities reflect, among other factors, degrees of autonomy and dependence. Interactions or practices are viewed in terms of three dimensions: communication, use of power, and sanctioning.

Social rules both govern and reflect the patterning of interactions and hence the continuity of social actions over time. Action always involves the practical intervention of actors into the physical or social world. Thus, actions produce outcomes which frequently represent transformations of social structure; in this sense social rules are always transformational.

Social resources are the vehicles or media whereby social structure is reproduced or transformed. Three structural dimensions are relevant in this process: signification, domination, and legitimation. Signification refers to the meanings of communication codes, expressed as signals, signs or symbols. Domination refers to command over persons (authorization) or over objects (allocation). Legitimation refers to the normative regulation of action.

Using these key concepts of social theory we propose a relatively simple framework of what may be considered important socio-structural conditions influencing health-related behaviours (Fig. 6.2), thus providing a preliminary answer to our first question.

We think the framework presented in Fig. 6.2 integrates the results of and the conclusions drawn from empirical research reviewed in the previous sections. Thus, *health-related rules* refer to specific patterns of preventive actions, of regular health-related practices and of coping behaviours. These behaviours were found to differ among social classes and to be associated with different health indicators. *Health resources* refer to the cognitive and normative elements associated with health-related behaviours (health culture) as well as the persons and collectivities involved (social network and social support). *Health motivation* refers to health-related needs or wants of individuals or to health-related goals shared by collectivities.

The framework can also be applied to provide a preliminary answer to our second question—how continuity of health-related behaviours over time is established or how behaviour changes are produced. Depending on the level of institutionalization, individual actors or collective actors (for example, the

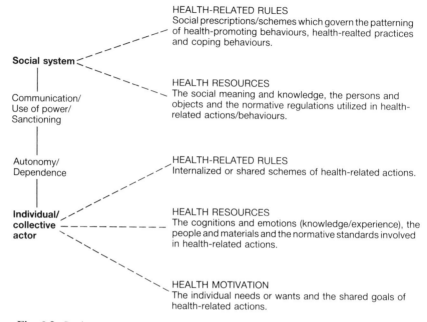

Fig. 6.2 Socio-structural and individual conditions of health-related behaviours.

family or other small groups) are influenced by the larger social system or they are autonomous in their health-related behaviours. Control or monitoring of such behaviours by the social system is seen to be achieved by three types of processes: communication, use of power, and sanctioning.

The individual monitoring of health-related behaviours, on the other hand, is accomplished by means of cognitive and emotional structures that represent the corresponding elements of social structure and that are internalized by individuals. Individual health-related action is further governed, or at least influenced, by factors that are unique to the individual actor—health motivations.

The cognitive, emotional, and motivational conditions of health-related behaviours are of course acquired or learnt structures. Depending on the social experience and on health experience they will be modified throughout the life cycle. Thus, the social system plays a double role in the structuring of health-related behaviours:

1. The social system helps to shape the individual conditions of such behaviours through 'health socialization'. This form of socialization must be assumed to be a life-long process of social learning and re-learning.

2. The social system influences health-related behaviours by means of social control such as communication, use of power, and sanctioning.

It is important, however, to note that this process is not unidirectional. Patterns of individual and collective health-related actions influence the social system continuously, either by stabilizing or by changing health-related rules and resources, which are defined to be key dimensions of social structure.

There are of course many open questions and a number of implications for future research. One example related to community-based prevention and health promotion programmes will suffice. Several such programmes have deliberately attempted to modify existing community structures, e.g. by reorienting health education and primary health care or by establishing new self-help activities. The available data on changes in cardiovascular risk factors, morbidity, and mortality indicates that community health promotion programmes 'can work' (Maccoby *et al*. 1977; Puska *et al*. 1985).

Unfortunately, in these projects and in several others under way, the community is treated as a black box and no changes in socio-structural factors are assessed (Maddox 1985). It is therefore suggested that in addition to changes in physiological and behavioural factors, changes in social health-related rules and resources also be evaluated. This would allow assessment of how far expensive long-term community programmes meet one of the major aims of the second revolution in public health, the modification of social environments.

References

Antonovsky, A. (1967). Social class, life expectancy and overall mortality. *Milbank Memorial Fund Quarterly* **45**, 31–73.

Antonovsky, A. (1981). *Health, stress and coping*. Jossey-Bass Publishers, San Francisco.

Antonovsky, A. and Shoham, I. (1978). *Social resistance resources and health in middle age*. Israel Institute of Applied Social Research, Jerusalem.

Benner, P. E. (1984). *Stress and satisfaction on the job, work meanings and coping of mid-career men*. Praeger Publishers, New York.

Ben-Sira, Z. (1985). Potency: A stress-buffering link in the coping–stress–disease relationship. *Social Science and Medicine* **21**, 397–406.

Berkman, L. F. and Breslow, L. (1983). *Health and ways of living. The Alameda county study*. Oxford University Press, Oxford.

Berkman, L. F. and Syme, S. L. (1979). Social networks, host resistance and mortality: a nine-year follow-up study of Alameda county residents. *American Journal of Epidemiology* **109**, 186–204.

Blaxter, L. M. (1985). Self-definition of health status and consulting reates in primary care. *Quarterly Journal of Social Affairs* **1**, 131–71.

Brown, G. W. and Harris, T. (1978). *Social origins of depression*. Tavistock Publications, London.

Buchmann, M., Karrer, D., and Meier, R. (1985). *Der Umgang mit Gesundheit und Krankheit im Alltag*. Haupt, Bern.

Cahalan, D. and Cisin, I. H. (1976). *Epidemiological and social factors associated with drinking problems*. Addison-Wesley, Reading, Mass.

Calnan, M. (1985). Research note, patterns in preventive behaviour: a study of women in middle age. *Social Science and Medicine* **20**, 263–8.

Cassel, J. (1974). Psychosocial processes and 'stress'; theoretical formulation. *International Journal of Health Services* **4**, 471–82.

Colerick, E. J. (1985). Stamina in later life. *Social Science and Medicine* **21**, 997–1006.

Doll, R. and Peto, R. (1981). *The causes of cancer*. Oxford University Press, New York.

Dressler, W. W. (1985a). Extended family relationships, social support and mental health in a Southern black community. *Journal of Health and Social Behavior* **26**, 39–48.

Dressler, W. W. (1985b). The social and cultural context of coping: action, gender and symptoms in a Southern black community. *Social Science and Medicine* **21**, 499–506.

Durkheim, E. (1897). *Suicide* (Translated in 1951 by G. Simpson). Routledge & Kegan Paul, London.

Folkman, S. and Lazarus, R. S. (1980). An analysing of coping in a middle-aged community sample. *Journal of Health and Social Behavior* **21**, 219–39.

Fox, A. J. and Goldblatt, P. O. (1982). *Longitudinal study: socio-demographic mortality differentials, 1971–75*, Series LS No. 1. HMSO, London.

Giddens, A. (1979). *Central problems in social theory*. Macmillan, London.

Goldberg, D. and Huxley, P. (1980). *Mental illness in the community*. Tavistock, London.

Gove, W. R. (1984). Gender differences in mental and physical illness: the effects of fixed roles and nurturant roles. *Social Science and Medicine* **19**, 77–91.

Green, L. W. (1984). Modifying and developing health behavior. *Annual Review of Public Health* **5**, 215–36.

Haskell, W. L. (1985). Overview: health benefits of exercise. In *Behavioral Health* (eds J. D. Matarazzo, J. A. Herd, N. E. Miller and S. M. Weiss), pp. 409–23. John Wiley, Chichester.

Haynes, S. G. and Feinleib, M. (1982). Type A behavior and the incidence of coronary heart disease in the Framingham Heart Study. *Advances in Cardiology* **29**, 85–95.

Henry, J. P. and Stephens, P. M.. (1977). *Stress, health, and the social environment. A socio-biologic approach to medicine*. Springer, New York.

House, J. S., Wells, J. A., Landerman, L. R., McMichael, A. J., and Kaplan, B. H. (1979). Occupational stress and health among factory workers. *Journal of Health and Social Behavior* **20**, 139–60.

Hunt, S. M., McEven, J., and McKenna, S. P. (1985). Social inequalities and perceived health. *Effective Health Care* **2**, 151–60.

Janz, N. K. and Becker, M. H. (1984). The health belief model: a decade later. *Health Education Quarterly* **11**, 1–47.

Kandel, D. B., Davies, M., and Raveis, V. H. (1985). The stressfulness of daily social roles for women: marital, occupational and household roles. *Journal of Health and Social Behavior* **26**, 64–78.

Karasek, R. A., Russel, R. S., and Theorell, T. (1982a). Physiology of stress and regeneration in job related cardiovascular illness. *Journal of Human Stress* **8**, 29ff.

Karasek, R. A., Schwartz, J. and Theorell, R. (1982b). *Job characteristics, occupation and coronary heart disease*. Department of Industrial Engineering and Operations Research, University of Columbia, New York.

Klein, S. D. (1980). Class, culture and health. In *Maxcy-Roseman, Public Health and Preventive Medicine* (ed. J. M. Last), pp. 1021–1034. Appleton-Century-Crofts, New York.

Knowles, J. H. (1977). The responsibility of the individual. In *Doing better and feeling worse: Health in the United States* (ed. J. H. Knowles). Norton, New York.

LaRocco, J. M., House, J. S., and French, J. R. P. Jr (1980). Social support, occupational stress and health. *Journal of Health and Social Behavior* **21**, 202–18.

Maccoby, N., Farquhar, J. W., Wood, P. D., and Alexander, J. (1977). Reducing the risk of cardiovascular disease: Effects of a community-based campaign on knowledge and behavior. *Journal of Community Health* **3**, 000.

Maddox, G. L. (1985). Modifying the social environment. In *Oxford textbook of public health* (eds W. Holland, R. Detels, and F. Knox), pp. 19–31. Oxford University Press, Oxford.

McKeown, T. (1976). *The role of medicine*. Nuffield Provincial Hospitals Trust, London.

McQueen, D. V. and Siegrist, J. (1982). Social factors in the etiology of chronic disease: an overview. *Social Science and Medicine* **16**, 353–67.

Marmot, M. G. and Morris, J. N. (1984). The social environment. In *Oxford textbook of public health* (eds W. Holland, R. Detels and F. Knox), pp. 97–118. Oxford University Press, Oxford.

Matarazzo, J. D. (1984). Behavioral health: a 1990 challenge for the health services professions. In *Behavioral health* (eds J. D. Matarazzo *et al*.). John Wiley & Sons, New York.

Morris, J. N. (1979). Social inequalities undiminished. *Lancet* **i**, 87.

OPCS, Office of Population Censuses and Surveys (1984). *General household survey, 1982*. HMSO, London.

Pearlin, L. I. and Schooler, C. (1978). The structures of coping. *Journal of Health and Social Behavior* **19**, 2–21.

Puska, P., Nissinen, A., Tuomilehto, J., Salonen, T. *et al*. (1985). The community-based strategy to prevent coronary heart disease: Conclusions from the ten years of the North-Karelia project. *Annual Reviews in Public Health* **6**, 147–93.

Rose, G. A. and Marmot, M. G. (1981). Social class and coronary heart disease. *British Heart Journal* **45**, 13–19.

Rosenman, R. H., Bran, R. J., Jenkins, C. D., Friedman, M., Straus, R. and Wurm, M. (1975). Coronary heart disease in the Western collaborative group study: final follow-up experience of 8 1/2 years. *Journal of the American Medical Association* **233**, 872–7.

Rosenstock, I. (1966). Why people use health services. *Milbank Memorial Fund Quarterly* **44**, 94–127.

Seeman, M., Seeman, T., and Sayles, M. (1985). Social networks and health status: a longitudinal analysis. *Social Psychology Quarterly* **48**, 237–48.

Siegrist, J. (1984). Threat to social status and cardiovascular risk. *Psychotherapy and Psychosomatics* **42**, 90–96.

Slater, C. H., Lorimor, R. J., and Lairson, D. R. (1985). The independent contributions of socioeconomic status and health practices to health status. *Preventive Medicine* **14**, 372–8.

Theorell, T., Alfredsson, L., Knox, S., Perski, A., Svensson, J., and Waller, D. (1984). On the interplay between socioeconomic factors, personality and work environment in the pathogenesis of cardiovascular disease. *Scandinavian Journal of Work and Environmental Health* **10**, 373–80.

Thoits, P. A. (1982). Conceptual, methodological and theoretical problems in studying social support as a buffer against life stress. *Journal of Health and Social Behavior* **23**, 145–59.

Townsend, P. and Davidson, N. (1982). Inequalities in health: the black report. Penguin Books, Middlesex.

Verbrugge, L. M. (1985). Gender and health: an update on hypotheses and evidence. *Journal of Health and Social Behavior* **26**, 156–82.

Waldron, I. (1983). Sex differences in human mortality: the role of genetic factors. *Social Science and Medicine* **17**, 321–33.

Wüthrich, P. (1979). *Alkohol in der Schweiz*. Huber, Frauenfeld and Stuttgart.

7

Risk factors investigation of health behaviour: Hungarian experiences

MIHÁLY KÖKÉNY, ZOLTÁN AJKAY and ILONA BOGNÁR

Conceptual issues in health promotion

The terms 'health education', 'prevention', and 'life-style' have been used in the medical and academic professions for several decades. In Hungary, as in many other countries, they are now part of everyday language. The WHO term 'health promotion' has proved very difficult to translate into Hungarian. The notion of health promotion is not completely captured by any, or indeed all, of the above. The concept of health promotion considers all individual behaviours which preserve and promote health and the wider system in which the individual exists. In this definition health does not mean the absence of disease but a state of physical, mental, and social balance where the individual's outer and inner environments are in harmony. Consideration should be given not only to present health but to health in the future. Intuitively, health can be preserved by making the individual more robust, a strategy best left to evolution, or by reducing the risk factors which endanger health. The latter strategy is the subject of this chapter.

Some risk factors, such as smoking and drinking, are easily viewed as the responsibility of the individual. Similarly, there are risk factors inherent in the environment: pollution and noise, for example. This apparent distinction between individual risk factors and environmental or societal risk factors is superficial. Some examples illustrate the difficulty in differentiating between them. Whether one moves from the city to the green belt involves elements of personal choice and environmental constraint. In developing countries the consumption of clean water may be considered an issue of either environmental protection or of individual health behaviour. This example is paralleled by the issue of food preservatives in industrialized countries.

Health behaviour is also influenced by both the individual and society. This is the problem of double determination. At the most individualistic level there are biological characteristics which will influence life-style. Age, the nervous system, hormones, skills of reaction, basic level of health, tolerance, and temperament all contribute to a person's way of thinking and ultimately to health behaviour. The environment has relatively little effect on these characteristics. They exert a lifelong influence on reactions to health-relevant situations and events. The relative importance of any of these characteristics changes across the life span.

Other individual characteristics are influenced to a greater extent by the social environment. Patterns of behaviour, attitudes, and values may be learned, from the family or school for instance, and will be affected by social structure. Again, it is important to stress that the relative importance of sources of influence will change over the life span. The influence of society may be exerted through the flow of information. It is important to recognize that the content of this information and the processes by which it is disseminated are culture bound. In most societies, however, the mass media have an ever-increasing role to play in this process. The effect of the media is direct. Even where programmes are not aimed specifically at promoting health, we are provided with many role models, both good and bad, such as the television personality who smokes and sportsmen.

Society can influence an individual's thinking in a less direct way, by providing a set of shared values—an ideology. Whether a society promotes collectivism or individualism will affect thinking, decision making, and ultimately health behaviour. Social structure exerts its influence via the distribution of resources. In material terms it is easy to see that the level of wealth can influence the diet. The distribution of non-material social wealth must also be considered: social structure can determine access to knowledge, for example. The influence of social wealth is not over-riding. As biological and social scientists all over the world have pointed out, improved standards of living do not necessarily or proportionally result in healthier behaviour. This reaffirms the interaction of individual and societal factors influencing health behaviour.

Having stressed the importance for health promotion of reducing risk factors and discussed the problem of attributing risks to the environment or individual behaviour and the analogous problem of attributing the behaviour of the individual to societal or individual factors, we will now describe the major risk factors affecting the Hungarian citizen. These risk factors may be considered under the following headings.

Diet

In Hungary the traditional diet contains a lot of animal fats and cereals. The average energy intake is 13 450 kJ/day. This is unjustifiably high and as a result obesity is widespread. Promotion of healthy eating based on proteins has so far had little success.

Physical activity

Urbanization and technical developments have resulted in the destruction of many jobs which involved physical work. The number of people living in the countryside and working in agriculture has decreased dramatically. Conversely, sedentary jobs have increased. Leisure time is dominated by watching television and pursuits involving any physical activity are being neglected. This is even the case with young people.

Smoking and abuse of alcohol and drugs

Smoking is becoming ever more prevalent, particularly among women and industrial labourers. Consumption of alcohol is also increasing. However, in Hungary it is the excessive and needless use of prescribed medicines which presents the greatest danger. This passive consumption of drugs as a means of preserving health represents a severe threat to a large proportion of the population.

Hazards of the human environment: aggression, tension

Our society is by no means free of problems arising from the individual's drive to achieve. Where goals for achievement are unrealistic, as is often the case, a person will inevitably fail. Meeting with this failure can produce aggressive reactions and a great deal of stress. These individual reactions can have effects on others. At a concrete level high stress may lead to dangerous driving or overtly violent behaviour. More subtly, family or workmates may be forced to carry some of the psychological burden.

Environmental hazards

It has already been pointed out that the dividing line between risk arising from the environment and that rooted in individual behaviour is very blurred. For example, it is difficult to imagine any individual action being able to reduce the risk from air pollution. Such behaviour would need to aim to change legislation. Where environmental hazards are caused by others, as for non-smokers in the presence of smokers, social pressure may be brought to bear.

Perspectives on the development of risk

It is relatively easy to list risk factors. It is not so easy to describe how these risks become salient in particular societies for particular people at particular times. The mechanism of exposure to risk needs to be elucidated. We will consider historical, developmental, and socio-structural influences on the emergence of risk.

Historical influences upon patterns of exposure to risk

Whilst it is frequently the case that the same risks exist in all industrial countries, the pattern of these risks is shaped by history. A description of the events thought to have influenced the development of risk in Hungary follows. During the last century mid-eastern European countries underwent unique changes and experienced unique threats. Wars threatened the security of life and property. Society underwent major changes which put an end to social injustice.

In Hungary the years that followed World War II saw unprecedented social mobility. The reallocation of employment from agriculture to industry and the geographical migration involved in this urbanization, gave rise to a 'new intelligentsia' from worker peasant origin. Suddenly and dramatically there was greater freedom of choice for the individual. Family cohesion was destroyed by the migration as well as the differing social positions occupied by the different generations. Moreover, no precedent existed for a life style based on such individual freedom. Traditional family-based patterns of behaviour were no longer appropriate, yet there was no obvious replacement. Accompanying this social revolution came a moral revolution. Religion lost its dominance. New social norms which allowed for the freedom of the individual developed gradually.

During these times of change health and health behaviour were not a priority. The concept of health was intricately related to the ability to work. By the 1960s the changes in social structure were well established. Society now had to adapt to a rise in living standards. Motorization spread rapidly and working time became shorter. Yet again personal choice increased as life-styles became still more flexible. Decisions had to be made on how to spend this newly acquired leisure time: whether to buy a television set or a weekend resort house. This element of choice extended only so far and unfortunately constraints which eventually came to bear promoted an unhealthy life style. Pricing policies still favoured an unhealthy diet. Alcohol and tobacco were widely available and considered status symbols. The neglect of health issues inherited from the previous generation combined with increased personal choice served only to allow unhealthy life styles to gain ground.

The economy changed again in the late 1970s. Living standards stopped rising, incomes polarized, and it became possible for many to take on a second job. Many were faced with the choice to take on extra work, sacrificing leisure time to earn more money but thereby increasing living standards. For those adopting this course smoking and drinking increased. This was probably a result of increased stress. In the background there were state programmes aimed at promoting healthy behaviour. Through these the public became more aware of the role of risk factors in non-communicable chronic disease. These programmes tended to influence a small group comprising the well educated and these people endeavoured to take part in some physical activity, have healthier diets, and to stop smoking and drinking.

Developmental changes and risk

In the previous section we described historical influences on the pattern of risk factors within our particular society. The next consideration in elucidating the process of exposure to risk is to consider changes in the situation of the individual across the life span. We describe below some features of the life stages childhood, adolescence, and adulthood, which imply special risks and the implications of these features for health promotion.

The importance of the family in shaping and influencing behaviour is a special consideration in Hungary. Terms such as 'family policy', 'family therapy', and 'family care' capture this idea. They refer to attempts to influence the individual through the family. The family's influence is obviously greatest on the young child. It is through the family that the child learns the concept and the value of health, patterns of living and personal hygiene, and times for eating and sleeping. The child learns not only from explicit instruction but from examples in the immediate social environment. Youth organizations report that the family rarely has a positive influence on children. Parents and grandparents living unhealthy lives are undesirable role models. A study of the family history of alcohol addiction and epidemiological studies of smoking show how unhealthy behaviour spreads like 'family contact infections'. It is currently the norm to allow an occasional drink or smoke on holiday. This approval serves only to make these health-damaging substances symbols of status—of being grown up.

An unstable family background may be seen as a risk factor since it often produces stress and emotional difficulties. The number of divorces is ever increasing. As previously suggested, in Hungary the traditional family structure is in disarray. The majority of families are incomplete. A fall in the number of children in a family along with increased mobility makes it ever more unlikely for three generations to live together. The health education provided by the family is becoming increasingly one-sided. Grandparents could play an important role in health education but this is rarely possible. The almost full-scale employment of women also affects the educational possibilities within the family. Increased living standards have increased the tendency to give children access to goods and habits which were never available to the parents. Many parents give their children too many sweets for example.

The biggest social influences in adolescence are the school and peers. It is unfortunate that in Hungary most of the secondary schools lack the facilities for promoting a healthy life-style: many find it difficult to provide good meals and sporting facilities. The value of secondary education is in general much neglected and inevitably the potential of these establishments for promoting health is for the most part ignored. The increased influence of peers is especially strong with respect to smoking and drinking. The social, emotional, and physical problems of adolescence should not be forgotten. Here exists an obvious source of stress. Other influences of these factors are not well expounded.

Throughout life the individual may be exposed to risk from chronic factors such as stress or acute life events, such as the loss of a partner. As a result of the demographic changes mentioned above old age often brings the added risk of loneliness. Old age has its own critical life events such as retirement or the loss of a partner, along with physical changes such as the deterioration of the senses.

Socio-structural factors and risk

Implicit in the notion of a socialist society is the striving to allow people the freedom to develop to their fullest human capacity. Governments of such societies strive to ensure a level of material and social well-being for their citizens that spares personal resources for education and social co-operation. Maintaining this standard of living has certain implications. The economy must be supported by productivity and the material goods and values of a society have usually been protected by militaristic means.

Finding the balance between personal freedom, the need to work, and the need to protect represent the basic problem of socialist countries. Because of the geographical position of Hungary these issues are influenced by the political and economic behaviour of other societies. With foreign trade undermining Hungary's economy and spiralling world armament, social issues are much neglected.

Although we have already suggested that historical events of the 1950s brought social issues to the fore, the resultant changes in the macrostructure did not always benefit the individual. Economic changes have already been shown to promote risk-taking by allowing individuals to overwork to improve their finances. Risky manual work is better paid than intellectual work. Groups such as large families, retired people, and young people are at greatest risk economically as well as psychosocially. In Hungary the fragility of material security is compensated to a large extent by social security which exceeds that of Western European countries.

All these macro factors have an influence on individual patterns of behaviour—whether this influence be conscious or unconscious. Unfortunately their combined effect works against social interest. Self assertion and material wealth are the major motivations of the individual and the family as the economic system favours those devoting their energies to material gain. The favoured political ideal of a person working for the whole society cannot compete with this reality. Stemming from this phenomenon of overworking to increase income and living standards, materialism and selfishness may be regarded as risk factors by virtue of their stressful nature. With this trend of overwork, smoking and drinking have increased. Smoking and drinking are now acceptable not only at social functions but in working meetings also.

Whilst social policy changes have met with some success in promoting healthy life styles the forceful influence of economic policy on health behaviour must be acknowledged. Conscious pricing should promote healthy eating habits and discourage smoking and alcohol consumption. In Hungary fatty foods are still relatively low priced compared to healthy ones. Alcohol is still relatively cheap despite repeated price increases. Despite extensive recent developments few people have access to sporting facilities. Sports equipment is expensive.

Increasing urbanization and industrialization increase environmental risks for the whole population. Green areas are decreasing. The use of chemicals and increased production of air pollutants present an ever-increasing danger to air, soil, and water. State regulations aimed at controlling these cannot compete with the greater force of economic interests, although public opinion is beginning to put some pressure on the offenders.

Most state organizations undertake activities which have some relevance to health. The school and its role have already been considered. Social security in Hungary is a basic right of citizenship and does not require additional or optional expenditures from the individual. Social security expenditures are deducted from income by a central mechanism. This provision gives the population a considerable sense of security and serves to promote equity. There are, however, several dysfunctions associated with this system.

This guaranteed financial security provides resources for those actively endangering their own health. Social security also means that it is worth being ill; some asocial people will actually feign illness. There are many lucrative jobs for those on the sick list or those declared disabled. This attraction of illness may unconsciously influence health behaviour.

Public health services are currently caught in a vicious circle. Since services are free of charge they are very accessible and as such a high morbidity measured by number of consultations is constantly increasing. Public health administrators and doctors are becoming more aware that primary preventive measures should be taken to alleviate this burden on resources, yet cannot spare any resources to this end. Few health professionals presently have the appropriate skills or motivation for primary prevention. This lack of motivation is congruant with the fact that those working in primary prevention are undervalued in financial and status terms. Principles of traditional biological medicine and authoritarianism still dominate in medical education, slowing the spread of ideas of social medicine and how to influence life styles. Recently some doctors have become involved in specific health education programmes. The starting point of a no smoking campaign must be doctors who are seen to be non-smokers.

The influence of the mass media on health behaviour must also be considered. On the positive side it can infuence behaviour overtly by providing information, or covertly in its provision of certain role models. It would be naïve to argue that all the information transmitted by the media promotes health.

Eliminating risk factors

In this section we consider the tactics of intervention into the process of 'risk—being at risk—health damaging behaviour'. A national programme has recently been outlined which aims to reduce risk factors at a general level by attempting to influence health behaviour. One aspect of this programme is intervention at the level of the macrocommunity. The aim is to change existing social structures which promote unhealthy behaviour. It outlines the role to be played by schools, industries, factories, social security, public health, and the mass media. At this level it is hoped generally to reduce risk factors and/or to make people more aware of their existence. To prevent susceptibility to risk the programme focuses on microcommunities: the family dwelling communities and small working collectives. The methods are based on personal contact, aiming to influence the behaviour of the individual with respect to particular behaviours. For maximum impact interventions at the micro and macro levels must coincide.

Healthy nutrition

One intervention promoting healthy nutrition at the level of the macrocommunity must be a change in pricing policy. The reduction of excessive calorie intake can only be based on a well-founded price system. The frequent occurrence of mass catering facilities offers potential for another intervention at the organizational level. If healthy food is provided by these facilities, the taste of the public may be influenced appropriately. A successful intervention has been the state control of preservatives added to food. This has been achieved through legislation of the canning industry. At the level of the microcommunity, 'lipid clubs' have become well established. These clubs provide information and dietary advice to those with constantly high blood cholesterol levels.

Physical activity

In Hungary there exists a glaring contradiction in sports promotion. At the highest competitive level, Hungary has excelled. In terms of participation by the general public, Hungary's record is extremely poor. To remedy this, attention should be given to school physical education. Schools should promote participation in sports which can be continued into adulthood, drawing attention to the social rewards that can be gained through participation. That special facilities are required for some sports has been recognized and the state has taken measures to increase the availability of such facilities. At the community level, formation of sporting clubs is being actively encouraged.

Protection of the environment

Environmental protection has been a priority state programme for some time now. The declared intentions of this programme can only be fulfilled if economic interests are pushed aside. In Hungary the importance of agriculture makes protection of the soil and control of the use of chemicals a major issue. In fact these issues have received much consideration. This illustrates well the balance of economic and social policy issues involved in promoting health behaviour. At the micro-environmental level the main concern is the proliferation of housing estates over the last decade. These bring problems arising from architecture. Often such housing constitutes a monotonous environment and encourages isolation.

Smoking, alcohol and drug abuse, mental hygiene

These behaviours are seen as resulting from misadaptation to society. As such, interventions aimed at modifying them are required to penetrate culture and the psychology of the individual. Hungarian studies have shown that accessibility of drugs and alcohol facilitates the development of their abuse. The effects of legislative interventions aimed at making these substances less accessible are undisclosed. If the abuse of these substances is functional, allowing the individual to escape from the pressures of life for example, then making these substances inaccessible may only result in an increase in other health-damaging behaviours which serve the same function. It is possible that these behaviours could be more harmful and less easy to monitor or control. If the notion of these unhealthy behaviours as misadaptations to society is accepted, the attention must be focused on the state and social structures which play a part in the individual's adaptation to society.

SECTION C

National surveys of health behaviour

INTRODUCTION

John K. Davies

The four chapters presented in this section of the book give descriptions of surveys from Wales, Finland, Denmark, and the USA. Although all of the surveys reported are different in scope and purpose, for example Wales as part of the evaluation of a country-based health promotion programme, Finland as part of a series of six national surveys each with different objectives, Denmark as part of a series of surveys of self-care, and the USA as surveys of behavioural risk factors, nevertheless there are common factors which interlink them.

In all of these countries there is a conscious move towards health promotion and prevention. Therefore the necessary motivation is there to provide impetus for these surveys. For example in the USA there has been a dramatic increase in the involvement of state health departments in the behavioural risk factor surveys, from 2 states in 1981 to 28 states in 1982–3.

The necessary human resources and expertise must be available. In Finland a complex infrastructure of researchers has been in existence for some years. Multi-disciplinary teams of researchers are necessary as reported in both Finland and the USA.

Emphasis is given in the chapters to the need to consider the practical use of survey results to aid policy-makers and planners. The Finnish surveys were specifically aimed towards problem-solving and the achievement of specific goals. Researchers were aware of these objectives but ensured that scientific freedom was incorporated into their work. In the United States the clustering variable was seen, not only in assessing the total risk in the population, but also in helping with a better understanding of the social context of health behaviours, which was important for the planning of health education programmes. Both here and in Finland it was felt that these new sources of data should be marketed to motivate policy-makers to action.

In the Finnish surveys they had relied heavily on a conceptual framework based on illness models which they felt were easier to deal with conceptually and empirically. (They also report that research money is more likely to be available to study work under the disease-prevention model.) In the Danish surveys, Dean reports on the value of the life-style concept in emphasizing the clustering of behaviours, their interconnectedness and their links with cultural, social, and psychological factors. In examining the influence of health perceptions and beliefs on health behaviour, the role of social network variables, and the coping concept, Dean highlights the recent attention given to the interactive nature of these variables. For the United States Hogelin reports that their comprehensive data shows that health behaviours can and do cluster, and that they may well be mutually reinforcing. Dean identified discrete health-related practices as behavioural elements in a life-style which was shaped by certain individual and social situational variables. The latter she saw as more important in understanding behaviour than individual motivations, attitudes and values.

All four chapters refer to methodology. Dean in particular gives a case-study approach to social research by discussing her methodology in some detail. She feels that of all the various methods to obtain behavioural data the social survey was the best suited to study population patterns of health-related behaviour and the interactions among the influences on this behaviour, i.e. social, psychological, and situational influences. This view was reinforced by Hogelin's experience in the United States. Nutbeam, in the Welsh Heart Survey, reported extensively on the methodology adopted. He examined the measurement of health behaviour with particular reference to outcome evaluation designs. The evaluation of the Welsh programme was as much with the process of change as with the measurement of outcome. Nutbeam describes the new indicators developed as more appropriate to the needs of community-based programmes.

All of the surveys reported considered the practical aspects of survey work; they also all realized the need for better conceptual bases to the study of health-related behaviour.

8

Methodological issues in the study of health-related behaviour

KATHRYN DEAN

The purpose of this chapter is to discuss research on health behaviour as it applies to the subject of health promotion. The health-related behaviour of individuals is now recognized as an important factor contributing to the maintenance of health and the control of chronic disease. Numerous research investigations have found associations between individual behaviours and measures of health status (USDEW 1979; McQueen and Siegrist 1980; Berkman and Breslow 1983). This body of research findings has stimulated widespread interest in the concept of life-style, a subject which has become the focus of a large number of programmes directed towards improving the health of populations. The importance of these developments is seen in the fact that 'healthy life-styles' have become a core component of the WHO European Regional Strategy for HFA 2000 (World Health Organization 1985).

This chapter is concerned with research strategies used to study self-care behaviours, the health-related behavioural elements of life-style, in a Danish research project. The task assigned to me is to focus on methodological issues involved in the study of health behaviour. Since life-style has assumed so central a position in health promotion policies, programmes, and services, the conceptualization and operationalization of this subject are fundamental methodological issues in health behavioural research.

Life-style: a core concept of health promotion

The concept of life-style has often been used to refer to a few habits of daily living measured and discussed as essentially discrete unrelated behaviours. Or more correctly, research associating behaviours measured discretely (i.e. smoking, alcohol consumption, dietary habits, and exercise patterns) with mortality and morbidity has resulted in a tendency to combine a limited range of behavioural practices under the rubric 'life-style'. This reductionistic approach to the concept of life-style not only focuses attention on a limited number of practices, but also separates individual behaviours from the flow of daily routines and from their social and situational context. Certain practices are defined as damaging, and educational or professional interventions are designed to change these habits in individuals. This development, while it shifts the focus of health services and programmes somewhat from specific body organs and diseases to specific behavioural practices, still reduces and compartmentalizes both health and behaviour in such a way that the essential interconnectedness of the determinants of both the health of individuals and the public health is lost.

A reductionist approach to the concept of lifestyle, however, is not universally accepted. For example, in the Health Promotion Glossary (1985) of the health promotion programme of the WHO Regional Office for Europe, 'lifestyle' is conceptualized as: 'a general way of living based on the interplay between living conditions in the wide sense, and individual patterns of behavior as determined by socio-cultural factors and personal characteristics' (World Health Organization 1985).

In this conceptualization individual health practices are only an element of culturally- and socially-determined interpretations and behavioural reactions. They are inter-related with other habits and are involved in constant processes of interactions among influences which either reinforce or alter them. Life-style research then would focus on interactions among health-related behaviours and the interacting influences which shape and maintain or change behaviour that affects health. In operational terms discrete health-related practices of individuals are more appropriately defined as 'self care behaviours', while clustering of behaviours and their interactions with cultural, social, and psycho-social factors may more meaningfully be considered 'life-style'. In this conceptualization of life-style the emphasis is on interconnectedness. Concepts of cause and effect are replaced by a focus on interacting processes of influence. Health outcomes are not caused, in this model, by specific behaviours, nor are discrete behavioural habits separated from their influence on other behaviours or on their own perpetuation. Efforts to promote healthy life-styles must, to be effective, understand the complex nature of these interacting forces. The extent of this complexity presents a difficult challenge to researchers studying health-related behaviour.

Three classes of variables have been studied extensively in relation to health and/or health behaviour. The influence of health perceptions and beliefs on health behaviour, especially preventive health behaviour and the utilization of professional services, have been studied in multiple investigations (Becker 1974; Dean 1984).

A second major area of study has focused on social network variables. A large body of work documents the influence of social networks and lay referral on illness behaviour (McKinlay 1973; Chrisman and Kleinman 1983). More recently, studies have focused on direct and indirect influence of social support on measures of morbidity and mortality (Gore 1980; House 1981; Turner 1983). These bodies of work generally do not consider the intervening influence of health behaviour on health outcomes.

A third class of variables increasingly studied in relation to health and health behaviour is concerned with the concept of coping. Earlier work predominantly focused on coping resources such as ego strength or defence mechanisms has been supplemented by research on coping styles and patterns of behaviour (Menagan 1983).

For the most part, these three classes of variables are represented in separate bodies of literature. Those studies which have investigated the three types of variables in multivariate analyses of health behaviour have often used static analytic models looking at relative weights in approaches that tend to conceptualize the variables as competing influences rather than examining the way these variables interact to influence health and health behaviour. However, recent attention has been drawn to the mutual and interacting nature of these variables (Mechanic 1983; Dean 1986a).

The Danish self-care studies

In the Danish self-care project, discrete health-related practices are considered behavioural elements embodied in a life-style shaped by social, psycho-social, and situational variables. The theoretical framework of these studies then involves an environmental perspective emphasizing social situational influences on the behaviour of individuals (Dean 1980). Social and situational variables are seen as more relevant to understanding behaviour than individual motivations attitudes and values.

While it is true that the individual learns basic value and behaviour patterns in early childhood, when the individual leaves the primary group multiple associations and unstructured interactions present new and competing values. The values and behaviour patterns learned in childhood are supplemented with social interactions that change the meaning of early experience. Motivation does not mean simply the will or intention to practise health protective behaviours. It refers to the set of perceptions that affect behaviour by creating an understanding of what is possible, pleasing, rewarding, and appropriate (Dean 1986a).

Personal development involves situational adjustments. In order to understand behaviour we must study 'what there is in the situation that requires the person to act in a certain way or hold certain beliefs' (Becker 1964). The situational theoretical perspective is counter to theories which ascribe behaviour to personality components formed in childhood and those which see behaviour as rigidly controlled by an underlying system of values. These explanations of behaviour build implicitly or explicitly on an assumption that human beings are essentially unchanging, that any behavioural alterations are superficial and trivial (Becker 1960). The behaviour of each individual is shaped by early learning, group influences, habits of coping, options for coping, support resources, and stress burdens. It is the interactions among these variables that compose life-styles and determine its behavioural elements.

The situational theoretical perspective may be viewed as a form of 'theory as process' (Glaser and Strauss 1967). Using this perspective, alternative forms of health-related behaviour can be used to focus the comparative analysis of various combinations of life-situational variables. Based on this theoretical perspective, the self-care studies involve a data-based search for the combinations of variables which shape behavioural responses. They are therefore a form of grounded theory, an approach to theory development which uses the data of social research for the systematic discovery and modification of theory. The analysis is guided and directed without the constraint involved in the need to prove or disprove specific causal relationships.

The research designs and statistical models used in the Danish self-care studies have been directed towards understanding inter-relationships among the three classes of variables mentioned above as well as their relative and joint influence on self-care practices. Behavioural data may be obtained by analysing secondary data sources (consumption patterns, use of services, etc.), by observation studies in laboratory or small group settings, by case studies of individuals, or by survey studies of groups. The latter methodology, social survey research, is best suited to understanding population patterns of health-related behaviour and interactions among social, psycho-social, and situational influences on health and health-related behaviour.

The self-care project has consisted of three survey studies of population samples. In these studies self-care is defined as the range of activities individuals undertake to enhance and restore health, including decisions to do nothing, activities to promote health or treat illness, and decisions to seek support or care in lay or professional networks (Dean 1986b).

Methodological issues in research design and implementation

A major goal of research on self-care behaviour is to learn how social situational variables and personal characteristics of individuals inter-relate to influence behaviour. No single research methodology can achieve this purpose.

Building on the results of qualitative open-ended interviews and findings from the research literature mentioned above, the investigations discussed here have been designed to develop systematically a body of information where findings from each study are elaborated in the subsequent investigation. The first study consisted of a nationwide population survey using a self administered postal questionnaire to examine the range and relative proportions of self-care responses to common illness conditions in the adult Danish population (Dean 1980; Dean *et al*. 1983).

The second survey was an interview investigation of a geographic sub-sample of the national survey respondents designed to study the influences of social support, coping and health belief variables on smoking habits, alcohol consumption, and self care responses to all illness episodes reported for a six-month period (Dean 1984, 1986a, 1988). The interviews were conducted in two confined geographical areas chosen to represent the range of residential areas and population density: the north-east areas of Zealand, including the capital city and its suburbs, and the north-east areas of the peninsula of Jutland, which includes the largest provincial city, small towns, and rural communities.

The third study conducted with a random sample from a small city and its surrounding rural areas examines the influence of social situational and attitudinal variables on health-enhancing, as well as illness-related, self-care behaviour in three age groups: 45–59, 60–74, and 75 years of age and older. This interview study was conducted in a community of 30 000 inhabitants which includes a mix of urban, suburban, and rural living arrangements.

In order to focus the remaining discussion of methodological issues in the study of health behaviour, three components of the research strategy which involve major methodological problems affecting the quality of the findings will be taken up: sampling, data collection, and the selection of a statistical model for analysing the data.

Sampling

Obtaining representative samples of general populations is a pre-requisite for valid analyses of interactions among variables thought to influence behaviour and for statistical inference to populations. Sources of error which can bias the findings of survey studies arise both from improper sampling procedures and from errors of measurement. Errors of the former type frequently result from weaknesses in the selection frames (sampling lists) available, or from the improper use of frames (Kish 1965).

The Danish National Population Register provides a selection frame which promotes the reduction of sampling error. It is possible when sampling from the register to narrow the study population in accordance with the goals of the investigation. In this instance all non-Danish residents of Denmark could be excluded from the study population in the interests of controlling for cultural differences which could not be validly studied due to inadequate representation of non-Danish cultural groups in the sample and the already complex research design. The studies in the project then examine social situational and attitudinal influences within the Danish culture. Cross-national investigations will study the effects of cultural differences on self-care.

Findings from methodological investigations show that individuals give less valid and reliable information when reporting for others (NCHS 1965b). Therefore children and the most elderly segment of the population were excluded. The national survey population thus consisted of all Danes between the ages of 18 and 78 years of age who resided in Denmark in the winter of 1978. A random sample of the study population was obtained by developing an extraction formula for drawing the sample which excluded all persons who:

- were not Danish citizens,
- were not alive at the most recent update of the register,
- had immigrated,
- were living in Greenland,
- were born before the year 1900,
- were born after the year 1959.

Once these criteria had been incorporated into the formula, the sample was generated by choosing a random date and selecting a number, corresponding to the appropriate sample size, of the persons in the study population born on that date. In the design of a survey investigation and the determination of a sampling procedure it is necessary to balance the survey objectives with the costs of various alternatives. This selection procedure is generally used in order to avoid prohibitive sampling costs. No biasing effects have been found from using this sampling procedure in Denmark.

A sample size of 1800 was determined by utilizing a formula for N in sampling for proportions. In this procedure a 95 per cent confidence limit and a 0.02 precision level were considered sufficient for the purpose of the study. The degree of precision used in determining the sample size depends on the cost of the sample relative to its value for the survey objectives. The goals of this study were to provide a baseline description of self-care behaviour in the Danish population and to obtain information on social and demographic variables that may influence self-care behaviour rather than to determine incidence or prevalence of the conditions studied. Additional costs of achieving greater precision were not warranted. However, in anticipation of non-respondents, particularly those in the oldest age category, it was decided to obtain about 2200 potential sample members in the sampling procedure.

A smaller sample was necessary for the second study, the purpose of which was to study interactions among situational and attitudinal variables. Since the sample members were respondents from the randomly selected national survey sample, the principal concern was to pick geographic areas which represented major differences in types and density of Danish communities. A sub-sample of 450 persons living in the two geographic areas described above was selected from national survey respondents.

A decision was made to aim for a sample of 450 to 500 persons in the study of three age groups over 45 years of age in a local community. The population register was again used to obtain a random sample of the selected community.

The rate of return is an important factor influencing the extent to which the goals of a survey research study are achieved. Of the 2203 persons thought to have received the questionnaires in the national survey, 1462 useable questionnaires were returned. Thus the final clean data set is based on information corresponding to a response rate of 66.4 per cent.

The most important question for the purpose of this study is not whether there is an over- or under-representation of certain types of persons in the sample, but whether or not any bias that may exist affects the direction of relationships. In a methodological investigation of the effects of non-response, Suchman (1962) found that in over 100 correlations little or no change occurred in the relationships, despite the fact that all of the correlations involved at least one variable which showed a difference in the marginal frequency distribution of the respondent and non-respondent groups.

Nevertheless, the effects of non-response are important to consider in order to assess potential sources of bias in the interpretation of findings. It is thus necessary to examine the characteristics of the respondents in relation to those of the study population. The national survey sample was representative of the age, sex, and marital status distributions of the population. It was as expected in survey studies using self-administered postal questionnaires, biased towards more educated persons (Dean *et al*. 1983).

The response rate in the area sub-sample was over 92 per cent. This is not surprising given that the persons contacted were respondents from the earlier study. Thus the most serious problem is the educational bias resulting from a sample based on persons responding to a mailed questionnaire.

The response rate and characteristics of the local community sample, N = 465, are presently being examined.

Data collection

Survey data may be obtained by self-administered questionnaires, by structured or open-ended interviews, or by a combination of these methods. Only the combination of approaches in studies which replicate and build on findings of other investigations can build a body of knowledge about health-related behaviour and how it affects health. The studies in this project have attempted to gain from the advantages of these different methodologies in order to establish a data base of information on relationships among social support, coping, health beliefs, and self-care variables.

The first survey obtained baseline information on self-care responses to common illness in the general population, using postal questionnaires to collect the data. The impersonal nature and standardized wording of mailed questionnaires, along with careful pre-testing of the data collection instrument, can increase the uniformity of the measurement situation. Another advantage of self-administered questionnaires is the reduced need for a quick response. This is particularly important in the collection of behavioural data when memory is a vital factor. The possibility to consider the response without any feeling of time pressure has been shown to increase the accuracy of the data obtained. (NCHS 1965b; Berkman and Breslow 1983).

By contrast, in interview investigations interviewer bias may enter the measurement situation in a number of ways. Differences among interviewers may affect both the type and amount of information obtained from respondents. In turn, interviewers may be affected differently by various types of respondents, changing the character of the interaction from situation to situation. Selective interpretation and recording of responses introduce another source of interviewer bias. Interview data may thus be less easily comparable than carefully standardized self-administered questionnaire data.

The data collected from self-administered questionnaires are, however, limited to what can be obtained from the written responses of the subjects. All efforts to enhance motivation and to stimulate memory must be incorporated into the cover letter, the research instrument, and the instructions for its completion prior to mailing the materials.

The research instrument

The limitations of a particular methodology may be modified by the construction of the research questionnaire. For example, standardization of the content of questionnaires help to ensure the validity and reliability of the findings. Framing questions in different terminology or alterations in the sequence in which questions are asked can influence their meaning. The accuracy of retrospective morbidity and behavioural data has been found to vary directly with the precision of survey questions (NCHS 1977; Kirscht 1971).

On the other hand, open-ended questions have the advantage of collecting data from respondents' perspectives, obtaining unexpected information and interesting quotes. Thus they are particularly useful for the collection of information in exploratory studies of subjects about which little is known.

These advantages have corresponding disadvantages. Open-ended questions require the recall of information with a minimum of stimulating cues. Data obtained from open-ended questions are difficult to code and often unreliable. Too much rapport, as well as too little, in an interview situation can seriously affect the accuracy of the data. Additionally, greater motivation is needed from both the interviewer and the interviewed to achieve reliable and unbiased outcomes.

Developing coding procedures for data from open-ended questions is extremely difficult since the need for new response categories can arise potentially at any stage of the coding. Additionally the judgement factor involved in categorizing open-ended data seriously affects the reliability of the findings. Ideally all open-ended data would be coded only by the principal investigator in order to achieve consistent judgement and reliable assignment of the responses to categories.

The range and richness of findings are of course the major advantages of open-ended data. These advantages can be incorporated into structured research instruments by building on the findings of qualitative studies or pilot interviews. The self-care survey questionnaires constructed on the basis of findings in the literature and information obtained in pilot interviews, utilized predominantly closed-ended questions. In addition to reduction of coder contamination, closed-ended questions enhance the comparison of all respondents on the same exact stimulus to reduce educational bias in the data. Some open-ended questions were used in the survey instruments when entirely structured questions could not obtain the information sought, for example medications used or advice given. So little is known about the range of behaviour which is considered health-enhancing by lay people that open-ended questions were also used regaring this subject. The open-ended data were all coded by one carefully trained coder who worked on all three self-care surveys and/or checked by the principal investigator.

Time period for the data collection

One of the most difficult decisions to make in the design of population survey studies of behaviour which must rely on self-reports is the time period for which the data will be collected. The findings of a considerable body of methodological research into the problem of recall are now available (NCHS 1965b, 1977). It is reasonable to reach a number of conclusions about the wide discrepancies found between self-reports and independently-recorded information on a wide range of human behaviour (Dean 1980). The non-correspondence between respondent-reported information and independent written records has been found:

1. less a problem of memory loss than of stimulating recall,
2. essentially unrelated to the individual demographic characteristics of the respondents,
3. seriously influenced by the degree of embarrassment or threat felt by the respondent in connection with the behaviour in question,
4. seriously influenced by the impact of the event, that is the personal importance or significance of the experience to the individual,

5. less related to factors of information levels and attitudes of the respondents than to the interview interaction process.

Early investigations conducted under the auspices of the US National Center of Health Statistics into the accuracy of self- or family-reported morbidity and illness behaviour data, as compared with that obtained from medical records, found a large amount of non-correspondence between the two sources (NCHS 1965a). Findings such as these led many researchers to conclude that lay people could not be trusted to provide valid and reliable information regarding their health and behaviour. However, careful examination of the findings suggested possible explanations for the magnitude of the non-correspondence between lay and professional data sources:

1. Differences in the terminology used by lay and professional groups.
2. Problems of arbitrariness in the classification of conditions by the researchers.
3. Effects of modifying adjectives such as 'serious' or 'frequent' in the research instruments.
4. Possible errors in the medical forms.
5. Conditions classified as 'possibly chronic' which may have been non-chronic conditions for which the interview schedule was not designed to elicit reports.
6. Interview effects.

It may be that similar condescending attitudes and opinions regarding the knowledge and ability of lay people which sometimes characterize professional patient interactions and research on 'compliance' has affected researchers' interpretations of discrepancies between lay and professional data sources. For example, such discrepancies have often been ascribed to memory loss or other types of respondent failure.

Reviewing these issues Kirscht observed:

> The conclusion seems to be that survey responses are poor substitutes for physician diagnosed conditions or even general evaluations of health. Reports on the use of health services and other medically relevant actions appear to fare better, but their accuracy depends on the type of information and manner in which it is sought. Note the assumption here, in relation to diagnoses, that the physicians' assessment is the 'true' one, or, put more broadly, that current medical conceptualization of illness is valid. I pass over the data that seems to indicate substantial unreliability among physicians in looking at the same patient and problems inherent in attempts to examine a cross-section sample. (Kirscht 1971, p. 522).

A factor which received scant attention in the search for the respondent characteristics associated with poor reporting of health and illness information was the interviewer effect (Dean 1980). A pioneer study by Rice (1929), and investigations of interviewer effect in the ensuing years, have provided a body of information regarding various kinds of interviewer bias. At the same time, methodological investigations have not found evidence that respondent attitudes, motivation, perceptions, or informational levels are responsible for incompatibilities in data from different sources.

The empirical evidence available points away from respondent failure as the cause of discrepancies found in data from household interviews compared with data obtained from medical records. The effect of lapsed time on recall is still of course an important consideration in study design. Twelve months and six months were the two recall periods used to study the reliability of a self-administered medical questionnaire designed to collect medical history and diagnostic data from patients (Collen *et al.* 1969). Generally, however, in the collection of data on acute morbidity or the utilization of physician services a very short period has been considered necessary for the collection of accurate data. The US Health Interview Survey uses a two-week recall period (NCHS 1975). A two-week period for data collection was also used in an international study of medical care utilization (NCHS 1969), in a study of morbidity experience and medication behaviour in England (Dunnell and Cartwright 1972), and in a Norwegian study (Christie 1975) of medication behaviour.

A Danish Morbidity Survey (Lindhart 1960), however, using a one-month recall period, found a high degree of correspondence between morbidity reported in lay interviews and diagnoses reported by physicians. Agreement was found in 71 per cent of the cases. A new diagnosis was added to the information provided by the patient only 6.5 per cent of the time, and there was disagreement between the doctor and the patient in 6.2 per cent of the cases.

In the analysis of recall in a methodological investigation studying the accuracy of family reports of hospitalization data, those respondents who did report their hospitalization were asked for the month of discharge. Not only did 82 per cent correctly state the month, only 3 per cent were in error by more than one month. The degree of accuracy was as great for hospitalizations that occurred 45 to 52 weeks prior to interview as for those occurring in the week immediately preceding the interview. These findings indicate that the 'under-reporting' of health events in household surveys is not primarily a function of the respondents' inability to place the event in time (NCHS 1965b).

For purposes of these investigations it was important to select sufficiently long time spans for the respondents to have experienced sufficient illness for meaningful analysis of multiple influences. Yet the respondents would be asked to recall detailed information about their self-care behaviour. The selection of six-month and two-month (for the second interview study) recall periods were based on the need to balance these rather conflicting aspects of the problem.

It is possible that the six-month time period has reduced the reporting of some conditions, especially milder manifestations of the symptoms. However, the goal of these studies was not to obtain incidence data, but to study the behaviour. In order to accomplish this it was necessary to obtain information on a wide range of health and illness experience.

Statistical strategy for the data analysis

The analytic task faced in the self care studies involves sorting out the relationships among many complex variables to: (1) distinguish those variables exerting direct influence from those exerting indirect influence; and (2) determine the nature of the connections among the variables. Substantive and theoretical considerations provide the framework of the analysis, but the statistical models and methods must be capable of validly testing theoretical questions.

In these investigations a situational theoretical perspective is focused on three classes of variables: coping, social network/support, and health beliefs. Not only habits of coping, but opportunities for coping options had to be considered. Both the composition and quality of the social network had to be examined to sort out the meaning and importance of these variables. Generalized as well as illness-specific health beliefs and perceptions have been associated with health-related behaviours. This means that many complex variables had to be included in our analyses, placing rigid demands on the statistical methods.

The multi-variate analytic problems in the self-care studies like those in most health behaviour research involve a large number of variables which are predominantly qualitative, mostly binary or ordinary categorical variables. Analyses of large multi-dimensional statistical problems are often undertaken with methods based on the theory of normal distributions because it is the statistical model for which calculations have been made possible and for which useable standard programmes are available. The variables in most studies of health behaviour are, however, about as far removed from the basis of a normal distribution model as can be imagined.

The large number of qualitative and discrete variables in our studies present an analytic problem where the data should be represented in contingency tables. Furthermore, the research goal in these investigations is to study the interconnectedness of factors and processes shaping behaviour rather than to test a causal relationship or determine relative weights for variables associated with behaviour. The research questions of interest relate to interactions, joint influence, chains of influence and hidden relationships among self-care behaviours, social, psycho-social, and situational variables.

Thus a statistical strategy for the analysis of the data sets which could validly analyse the inter-relationships among many complex categorical variables was needed.

While the theoretical basis for the multi-variate analysis of contingency tables has been developing rapidly in recent years (Bishop *et al*. 1975; Anderson 1984; Edwards and Kreiner 1983), technical advances for this type of analysis are still extremely limited. One can, depending on financial and time constraints, work with at best 7–10 dimensional contingency tables using the standard programmes now available. However, the only way one can reach reasonable certainty that the conclusions regarding interactions among a given number of variables are logically tenable is by analysing them together in the same model. If the marginal conclusions can be seen as necessary consequences of the complete model, there is a logical consistency in the results. If the marginal results cannot be derived from the analysis of the unified complete model, there is a break in the logic of the conclusions.

Thus, the practice in complex multi-variate statistical problems of conducting contingency table analyses on the basis of generally available programmes, i.e. some of the variables at a time, presents problems when the researcher wants to generalize results from the marginal analyses to conclusions regarding the total large dimensional model (Simpson's paradox discussed in David 1979). Even though the sub-analyses individually may be considered to have superficial meaning they will usually result in contradictory and inconsistent results. Only if the combined marginal conclusions can be seen as necessary consequences of the complete model can they be considered logically valid results.

The statistical strategy used for the analysis of data in the self-care project is based on the over-riding demand that all sub-analyses lead to a unified model for the complete large dimensional frame of reference. The conclusions are based only on that complete model and all marginal analyses must be derived from and consistent with the total model. The methods used in the strategy are based on graph mathematical theory, developed in a sub-class of log-linear models for contingency tables (Darroch *et al*. 1980; Edwards and Kreiner 1983).

Since the complete model cannot be analysed in a single procedure, and the marginal results cannot automatically be generalized to the complete model, the strategy is based on a running control of the complete set of variables which form the model. These model-checking procedures assume a central place in the strategy for a valid analysis of our complex multi-variate research problems.

In the first step of the strategy, a screening of the data is conducted using hierarchical, log-linear models for contingency tables to select and improve a practically usable base model which can provide the starting point for the core analysis; that is, for the analysis which tests the substantive and theoretical research questions of interest in the investigation.

The screening determines if the large dimensional table is validly collapsible in the context of the theoretical and substantive research questions of the study and which marginal relationships must be considered in the specific analyses.

The three essential components of the strategy are:

1. That all aspects of the analysis are directed towards formulating a unified model for the total large dimensional table.
2. That a graph theory analysis of the interaction graph is conducted.
3. Careful control of the base model generated by the graph analysis to assure a valid foundation for the testing of the theoretically determined research questions.

In the testing of substantive or theoretically based research questions, the structure of the base model must always guide the analysis. This is the case regardless of the collapsibility of the structure of the model. While the goal is to simplify the structure of the data, *when the structure remains complex, this complexity must be recognized in the testing of research questions*.

Conclusion

The findings from our analyses to date suggest that the way illness is experienced (perceptions regarding the seriousness of symptoms and perceived health status) is a pathway through which causal factors shaping self-care behaviour operate. Variables representing stressful life situations, social support and habits of stress reduction appear to be major forces interacting to shape self-care behaviour. Generalized health beliefs appear to operate as a supplemental influence affecting health behaviour.

It is emphasized that the interactions and joint influences are complex. For example, psycho-social support has emerged as an important variable related to morbidity and mortality. The analyses of these Danish data sets suggest that social support plays an important role in self-care behaviour as well. Family structure, the number of adults living in the household and satisfaction with or the adequacy of the social support provided by the personal social network were all related to whether or not symptoms were interpreted as serious, the proximate determinant of self-care behaviour. Habits of coping with stress and faith in the ability of medical care to protect or restore health also influenced the symptom perceptions. Put another way the symptom perception variable collects joint effects of interactions among social and psycho-social influences that shape illness behaviour.

Persons who usually discuss their problems with others in their social network, and those who find ways to rest and relax when feeling stressed, reported serious symptom episodes considerably less often than persons who attempt to reduce stress by taking medications or trying to forget their problems. Similarly, persons with high confidence in their own capacity to influence health reported less serious symptom episodes. On the other hand, strong beliefs in the capacity of the medical science to protect health was associated with more serious illness episodes.

Persons who discuss their non-medical problems with their doctors had different self-care patterns of response independent of the type of symptoms or the perceived seriousness of the illness episode. An exploration of the possibility that this finding may represent available social support in the social network revealed that persons who discuss non-medical problems with doctors more often reported insufficient or non-supportive social relationships. These persons in turn had generally passive patterns of self-care behaviour, consulting doctors for all types of symptoms and more often using medicines to treat illness episodes.

The joint and interacting influences of the coping, social network/support, and health belief variables on health maintenance aspects of self-care are now being analysed in the data from the third self-care investigation.

In the three studies of self-care behaviour discussed in this chapter, an attempt has been made to build on the findings of each investigation in a process of developing a knowledge base of the range of health-related behaviour and the interacting processes shaping it.

The methods available to survey researchers all have advantages and disadvantages. In the self-care studies we have used a range of methods in an attempt to gain from the advantages of different methodologies. Of course using different methods cannot alone assure the validity of findings. The assumptions inherent in the theoretical perspective must be clearly addressed. Not only the validity of the items and scales measuring concepts, but also the logic of the research design and the ability of the statistical models to validly test the research questions of interest, determine the quality of the findings.

It may be concluded from both the findings of the first two studies and the preliminary results of the latest investigation, that individual self-care practices are not discrete independent behaviours which can be separated from their social and situational context. Patterns of self-care behaviour interacting with social and situational influences form life styles. Health-enhancing life styles will not be achieved by focusing on individual behaviours separated from their social and cultural meaning.

References

Anderson J. A. (1984). Regression and ordinal categorical variables. *Journal of the Royal Statistical Society* **B.46**, 000.

Becker, H. (1960). Notes on the concept of commitment. *American Journal of Sociology* **66**, 32–40.

Becker, H. (1964). Personal change in adult life. *Sociometry* **27**, 40–53.

Becker, M. (1974). *The health belief model and personal health behavior*. Slack Press, Thorofare, NJ.

Berkman, L. and Breslow, L. (1983). *Health and ways of living*. Oxford University Press, New York.

Bishop, Y., Fienberg, S., and Holland, P. (1975). *Discrete multivariate analysis: theory and practice*, The MIT Press, Cambridge, Mass.

Chrisman, N. and Kleinman, A. (1983). Popular health care, social networks and cultural meanings: the orientation of medical anthropology. In *Handbook of health, health care and the health professions* (ed. D. Mechanic). The Free Press, New York.

Christie, V. (1975). Social status og Bruk av Vitamin preparatir, jernpreparater og Medikamerter [social status and the use of vitamin, iron and psychotropic preparations]. *Tidskr. Nord. Saegeforen* **95**, 1216.

Collen, M., Cutler, J., Siegelabu, A. B., and Cello, R. (1969). Reliability of a self administered medical questionnaire. *Archives of Internal Medicine* **123**, 664–81.

Darroch, J., Lauritzen, S., and Speed, T. (1980). Markov fields and log linear interactions model for contingency tables. *Annals of Statistics* **8**, 522–39.

David, A. (1979). Conditional independence in statistical theory. *Journal of the Royal Statistical Society* **B44**, 1.

Dean, K. (1980). *Analysis of the relationships between social and demographic factors and self-care patterns in the Danish population*. Ph.D. thesis. University of Minnesota.

Dean, K. (1984). Influence of health beliefs on lifestyles: what do we know? *European Monographs in Health Education Research* **6**, 127–51.

Dean, K. (1986a). Self-care behaviour—implications for aging. In *Self care and health in old age* (ed. K. Dean, T. Hickey and B. Holstein). Croom Helm, London.

Dean, K. (1986b). Lay care in illness. *Social Science and Medicine* **22**, 275–84.

Dean, K. (1988). Social support and health—pathways of influence. *Health Promotion*, forthcoming.

Dean, K., Holst, E., and Wagner, M. (1983). Self care of common illness in Denmark. *Medical Care* **21**, 1012.

Dunnell, K. and Cartwright, A. (1972). *Mechanic takers, subscribers and hoarders*. Routledge and Kegan Paul, London.

Edwards, D. and Kreiner, S. (1983). The analysis of contingency tables by graphical models. *Biometrika* **70**, 553–565.

Glaser, B. and Strauss, A. (1967). *The discovery of grounded theory*. Aldine Atherston, Chicago.

Gore, S. (1980). Stress buffering functions of social supports—an appraisal and clarification of research models. In *Stressful life events and their contexts* (eds B. S. Dohrenwend and B. P. Dohrenwend). Prodist, New York.

House, J. (1981). *Work, stress and social support*. Addison-Wesley, Reading, Mass.

Kirscht, J. (1971). Social and psychological problems of surveys on health and illness. *Social Science and Medicine* **5**, 519.

Kish, L. (1965). Survey sampling. John Wiley and Sons, Inc., New York.

Lindhardt, M. (1960). *The sickness survey of Denmark 1951–1954*. Munksgaard, Copenhagen.

McKinlay, J. (1973). Social networks, lay consultation and help-seeking behaviour. *Social Forces* **51**, 375.

McQueen, D. and Siegrist, J. (1980). Social factors in the aetiology of chronic disease—an overview. *Social Science and Medicine* **16**, 353–69.

Mechanic, D. (1983). The experience and expression of distress: the study of illness behaviour and medical utilization. In *Handbook of health, health care and the health professions* (ed. D. Mechanic). The Free Press, New York.

Menagan, E. (1983). Individual coping efforts: moderators of the relationship between life stress and mental health outcomes. In *Psychosocial stress* (ed. H. Kaplan). Academic Press, New York.

National Center for Health Statistics (1977). *A summary of studies of interviewing methodology* (Vital and Health Statistics, series 2, vol. 69). U.S. Government Printing Office, Washington, D.C.

National Center for Health Statistics (1975). *Acute conditions incidence and associated disability* (Vital and Health Statistics, series 10, vol. 102). U.S. Government Printing Office, Washington, D.C.

National Center for Health Statistics (1969). *International Comparisons of medical care utilization: a feasibility study* (Vital and Health Statistics, series 2, vol. 33). U.S. Government Printing Office, Washington, D.C.

National Center for Health Statistics (1965a). *Health interview responses compared with medical records* (Vital and Health Statistics, series 2, vol. 7). U.S. Government Printing Office, Washington, D.C.

National Center for Health Statistics (1965b). *Comparison of hospitalization reporting in three survey procedures* (Vital and Health Statistics, series 2, vol. 8). U.S. Government Printing Office, Washington, D.C.

Rice. S. A. (1929). Contagious bias in the interview. *American Journal of Sociology* **35**, 420.

Selltiz, C., Wrightsman, L., and Cook, S. (1976). *Research methods in social relations*. Holt, Rinehart and Winston, New York.

Suchman, E. (1962). An analysis of 'bias' in survey research. *Public Opinion Quarterly* **26**, 102–111.

Turner, R. (1983). Social support and psychological distress. In *Psychological stress* (ed. H. Kaplan). Academic Press, New York.

U.S. Department of Health, Education and Welfare (1979). *Healthy people: the surgeon general's report on health promotion and disease prevention*. Background Papers, U.S. Government Printing Office, Washington, D.C.

World Health Organization (1985). *Health promotion glossary*. Health Promotion Unit, WHO Regional Office for Europe, Copenhagen.

9

Health-behaviour measurement in the evaluation of community-based health-promotion programmes—A case study: the Welsh Heart Programme

DON NUTBEAM

Introduction

Community-based demonstration programmes such as the Welsh Heart Programme may be seen as having three essential evaluation goals, namely:

- To develop and test the *effectiveness* of programmes in improving the health of individuals and communities both by maximizing health-enhancing factors and reducing health risks. These may be related to individual life-styles or the environments in which people live and work. Relative costs of alternative approaches might also be considered here, along with the monitoring of any indirect benefits and negative effects.
- To test the *feasibility* of implementation, and within that the *acceptability and uptake* of programmes by individuals and communities who participate in their development and implementation.
- To test the *generalizability* of programmes, and their potential for replication in a range of different settings, geographical areas etc. This enhances the relevance and usefulness of programmes for policy makers. Cost is again an important factor here, together with negative effects and indirect benefits.

In the first case the main emphasis is on measuring the *outcome* (or end points) of implementation activity, in the second and third it is on the *process* (or mechanics) of implementation. Such 'process evaluation' would also include an assessment of impact (i.e. penetration) of the programme. It should be stressed that all three goals are closely inter-related. This chapter considers the use of health behaviour measurement in this evaluation process with particular emphasis on its role in outcome evaluation.

Outcome evaluation design

Before specific consideration can be given to the role of health behaviour measurement in evaluation it is important to provide an overall context through a more general discussion of evaluation principles. A logical sequence for tackling a public health problem would involve the field testing of hypotheses and methods first developed in tightly controlled, usually small group studies. However, while such randomized controlled trials are recognized as one of the more powerful tools in science, their relevance and practical usefulness in community-based health promotion studies is limited. The selection process used in such studies, and the artificial environments in which the study is confined, usually minimizes their relevance to 'real-life' community settings, and thereby limit their generalizability. They are also extremely expensive when applied to large numbers of people.

The field nature of a community demonstration programme denies the experimental control of many variables. Communities are complex and changing systems. People move in and out of communities, thus diluting the impact of planned social change. Unpredicted events (such as unemployment related to a decline in one particular industry) may affect a single community in ways not shared by another under study. There are logistical problems which place constraints on communication and stretch available resources. Perhaps most important of all, the causal chain in a community system is longer and harder to trace than in a clinical research study on volunteers. For example, diffusion effects and interaction among varied inputs are far more likely to occur in a community system. Freedom to select programme implementation areas randomly is also limited. This is not only by geographical influences (for example, shared media) but by ethical, practical, and political considerations associated with the allocation of limited resources. For these reasons it is not possible to test specific epidemiological or behavioural hypotheses in the kind of community demonstration programme represented by the Welsh Heart Programme.

However, community programmes offer far greater potential cost-savings simply because they deal with larger numbers of people and draw upon the existing resources of the community. In this sense they can provide policy-makers with information more relevant to their problems than that obtained from tightly controlled research in an artificial environment. A quasi-experimental evaluation design is more appropriate for community-based studies, based on 'pre and post' tests to measure change in communities where interventions are not randomly allocated but a reference or 'control' population is used. This reference population is normally matched in terms of size and demographic characteristics, but separate geographically from the programme implementation area. It provides the important comparison point for detecting net change. The Welsh Heart Programme has an external reference area, closely matched for key health, social and economic indicators. Life-style changes are being monitored in this region using the same methods as within Wales. However, the same problems associated with unpredictable events and complexity of analysis also apply in the reference area—hence its use alone in improving confidence is limited. However, improvements in the reliability of conclusions about cause and effect can be achieved in other ways:

- *Studying the process of change* in communities using techniques such as *network analysis* and *dose-effect measurement*. The former technique is used to trace the path of communications within a community, determining such issues as dilution or distortion of programme inputs, as well as their relative efficacy in achieving change. The experimental use of this technique is already under way within the Welsh Heart Programme. In the latter case it is possible to correlate differences in input directed towards different population samples, with effects on various dependent variables. Within Wales this technique is readily applicable as each of the Health Authorities is planning a different type of programme input, aimed at different population groups.
- *Analysis of unobtrusive measures of change.* The measurement of life-style change can be supported in an aggregate sense by monitoring changes in food purchase or tobacco sales as consistent with reported changes in diet and smoking. Arrangements have already been made with some of the major retailers in Wales and the reference area for this type of monitoring exercise.

These techniques, combined with a quasi-experimental study design, help to provide firmer evidence of cause-and-effect relationships in community-based programmes.

Appropriate indices for measuring change in community-based health-promotion programmes

Ultimately programmes such as the Welsh Heart Programme are intended to have a favourable impact on the incidence of heart disease—measured primarily in terms of a reduction in premature death or disability from coronary heart disease. Most other 'health' programmes are also funded in the belief that they will have a favourable impact on reducing disease and premature death.

However, achieving such changes through life-style intervention may take between 10 and 15 years to be reflected in disease rates. Most programmes are not funded to run for such long periods. The Welsh Heart Programme, for example, is funded for five years. Specific thought, therefore, has had to be given to which legitimate indices can be used as indicators of a successful outcome over five years.

A reasonable consensus of known risk factors for heart disease is available, summarized in the WHO Expert Committee Report on Coronary Heart Disease Prevention (WHO 1982). From this the Welsh Heart Programme has included the measurement of health behaviours such as smoking status, physical activity, diet, and alcohol consumption in the population, as well as the measurement of biological factors such as body mass, serum cholesterol, and blood pressure levels in the population. In addition, improvements in knowledge and understanding of risks to health as well as knowledge of appropriate life style changes are also essential.

The simple measurement of health behaviours as risk factors is not sufficient on its own. Most would agree that disease prevention is only one half of the desired outcome and that the promotion of positive health and well-being should be an important, if not the major goal of health programmes. In addition, considerable emphasis is also placed on achieving changes in the environment as an important strategy for supporting life-style change.

Unfortunately the difficulty of measuring personal characteristics such as self-esteem and health locus of control has resulted in the available literature being discounted as 'unscientific' in some circles. The substantial body of literature on stress is often considered in this category. There is, however, a considerable volume of published literature within the education and social science fields which shows the very close relationship between behaviour and personal beliefs, on the one hand, and the physical and social environment, on the other. If health behaviour is the 'acceptable' short-term index of achievement, then there is also good reason to include a wider range of factors closely associated with health behaviour in the short-term outcome evaluation.

Thus within the Welsh Heart Programme we have included simple measures of perceived health, health locus of control, and access to social support within our community survey work. The methodology employed to measure these factors and the health behaviours mentioned above is described in greater detail in the next section.

In addition, a separate community-based study concerned with detecting and measuring supportive changes at a macro-level, and within the environment, has also been established. Specifically four studies are under way, namely:

1. A study of changes in restrictions on smoking in public premises.
2. A study of changes in the availability of healthier food choices both in restaurants and other public catering establishments, and in work-place canteens.

3. A study of changes in the provision of and access to exercise facilities.
4. The monitoring of changes in food retail patterns and food supply.

The Welsh Heart Health Surveys

In order to assess changes in health behaviour and related factors the Welsh Heart Programme is carrying out a series of independent cross-sectional surveys of a random sample of the population in each of the nine health authorities in Wales. During the summer of 1985 the first of these surveys, providing baseline data, was completed. By repeating the survey in 1988 and 1990, changes towards specific targets can be assessed. Full details of the survey design and methodology are available separately so only a brief summary will be given here (WHP 1985b, 1986a).

In the 1985 survey the sample selection was based on households which were randomly selected from the electoral registers in Wales. A total of 21 650 households were contacted and 32 460 eligible (i.e. aged 12–64) participants were included. The first part of the study consisted of a short, household interview to obtain basic demographic details of individuals and the household. Participants were then given a comprehensive questionnaire for self-completion covering the full range of indicators required for the outcome evaluation. These include health behaviours such as smoking, food and alcohol consumption, and exercise participation; also knowledge and attitudes towards reducing the risk of coronary heart disease. In addition the other indicators concerned with perceived health, access to social support and locus of control were also included. Reported angina and respiratory symptoms, and previous diagnosis of hypertension and myocardial infarction, were also assessed through questionnaire. The response rate for household interview was 94 per cent, and self-completion booklet response was 68 per cent overall, ranging from 72 per cent to 64 per cent between health authorities. Two studies have examined the possible non-response bias to the self-completion questionnaire. The first, an analysis of demographic data available from the household interviews (which included the total sample), showed that slightly more women than men responded, less younger adults (under 35) responded than older, and a higher proportion of social class I, II, and IIIN responded than classes IIIM, IV, and V. However, the second study, based on personal interviews with a representative sample of 200 non-responders, indicates that those responding are representative of the total population and that non-response bias is minimal.

Two thousand of this population, randomly selected from 15 600 volunteers, were offered a follow-up clinical examination which was used to validate self-reported behaviour and to provide additional data on blood lipids, blood pressure, and cardiovascular fitness.

In many cases, questions used in the survey are the same or comparable to other studies being conducted in the UK and abroad. Where relevant the data obtained through clinical examination has been collected and analysed according to MONICA protocol and thus should also be comparable.

The sample size was determined according to a standard formula for community studies, and structured so that each of the nine health authorities has a minimum sample of 2000 regardless of absolute population size. This allows for quite small changes in health indicator means to be detected on an all-Wales adjusted basis. At local health authority level a minimum sample of 2000 has provided a reasonable data-base for local communities to plan their own specific programmes, and will be sufficiently large to identify changes in health behaviours between authorities (further details of the assumptions made are available in the survey protocol). This will then allow for comparison between the different types of intervention which will be conducted in the different authorities. It should be emphasized that such comparisons cannot be used for assessment of achievements between health authorities because of the confounding nature of uncontrolled variables. However, network analysis and dose–effect correlations between authorities, combined with comparisons to the reference area, will enable a more confident comparison of effects between different types of interventions.

An area in England carefully matched for age, sex, and socio-economic status, employment structure, and heart disease mortality, has been chosen for the reference area (further details are available in the survey protocol). The baseline survey was conducted in this area at the same time with strict adherence to identical methodology and sampling procedures. No clinical examinations were conducted there. The results from the survey are available in a series of reports published by the Welsh Heart Programme (e.g. WHP 1986b).

Thus, in summary, the outcome evaluation of the Welsh Heart Programme is based on the measurement of change in health behaviour indicators using a quasi-experimental evaluation design built on independent cross-sectional sample population surveys. This basic evaluation tool will be supported by the use of a reference population, along with additional studies of the process of change and unobtrusive measures of change. In addition supporting changes in the environment will also be monitored.

Process evaluation

The Welsh Heart Programme was established as a national demonstration project. As such, one major goal is to develop and evaluate different means of achieving change in life styles within a single region. Process evaluation is directed towards this goal by specifically examining the mechanism of change. It is intended to identify features of a project which enhance or hinder its chances of success as the project develops. This helps to influence the further development of the programme within the region and enables early feedback to others outside the study region. Process evaluation is particularly concerned with the feasibility, acceptability, and generalizability of defined approaches to achieving change, but also needs to address some of the reasons *why* and *how* people change health behaviour.

This aspect of evaluation of community programmnes has often been under-valued or presumed as serving only the needs of the outcome evaluation. Although success may have been achieved and carefully measured in programmes, unless attention is paid to the above issues once a project team withdraws from the study area the achievements may well decline. The identification and separation of component parts to the programme, and the life of the achievements beyond the work of the directorate, are thus essential evaluation issues which must be addressed.

Virtually all of the activities supported with resources by the Welsh Heart Programme will include some assessment of these important issues of feasibility and acceptability through stated objectives. More specifically, however, two research-based projects are planned to provide an overview on process evaluation and form an important link between the evaluation and programme development.

The first is a specific and structured attempt to test the response of the general population in Wales to the programme's various components—to identify some of the reasons why and how people change. In addition, this market resarch project is intended directly to involve the communities in Wales in the design and development of component projects of the Welsh Heart Programme. It is described in more detail below.

The second is a project intended to measure the level of support and involvement among some key opinion leaders in Wales. This is a specific study of health behaviour change among a potentially very influential group within Welsh society. An integral component will include an educational intervention based on the findings, intended to improve commitment to achieve greater practical support and resources for health promotion. The groups included in this study are general practitioners, nurses (both from hospital and community), teachers, journalists, and local politicians (including local councillors and health authority members). This is also described in more detail below.

Community monitoring panels

Consumer panels are widely used in the market research fields to pre-test the acceptability of new projects, or comment on proposed promotional campaigns. They are also used to monitor the impact of particular campaigns. This project is designed to adapt this simple research tool to provide a genuine structured mechanism for involving local communities in Wales in the development and monitoring of impact of the Welsh Heart Programme. It will also be used to inform programme directors on aspects of programme planning.

The present scheme is based on the recruitment of small groups of people from a small number of representative communities in Wales (e.g. a rural community, inner city community, mining community, Welsh speaking community, etc.). These meet at intervals, and are helped in group discussion by a trained facilitator. The focus of discussion is in part based on a semi-structured interview intended to identify what aspects of the programme, both national and local, had penetrated the local community, and what had been the response to it. The group might also then collaborate as a sounding board for new ideas and planned projects as a first stage in field testing. In both cases new ideas and suggestions from panel members are strongly encouraged. Because of the obvious 'training effect' of serving as a panel member there is a regular turnover of panel membership.

The Welsh Opinion Leaders' Health Study

This study focuses on some of the key groups in the community which play a crucial role in the implementation process, and in shaping the community's response to activities initiated through health promotion programmes. These groups include general practitioners, nurses, teachers, journalists, and local politicians (including local government representatives and health authority members).

To effect change requires action at all levels in communities. New life styles are innovations that diffuse with time through natural networks of the community. This diffusion occurs at a different rate in different groups (Rogers 1983). Health and education professionals, and other community leaders, have a unique role both as change agents (attempting to initiate the innovation—diffusion process) and opinion leaders (speeding up the process). They can particularly act as health advocates, drawing attention to the need for improvements in the wider environment which has such a powerful influence on health choices.

For these reasons the commitment and active participation of these groups is vital. For community-based programmes to be successful in the long term it is essential both to identify the present level of commitment of these opinion leaders, and to identify ways of improving this commitment and thereby gain a greater practical support and resources for health promotion. This is the dual purpose of the opinion leaders' study.

The study will be conducted through self-completion questionnaire, and by physical examination in a proportion of subjects. Changes in health behaviour, attitudes, and commitment to the aims of the programme, and work practice relating to the programme will be monitored over time in these groups. Special attention will be given to identifying ways in which commitment has been gained (or lost). The lessons learned through this study should provide important and generalizable practical guidance on involving health and educational professionals, and community leaders in health promotion programmes. It will also enable the monitoring of the acceptability of programme components to relevant groups.

Summary

The Welsh Heart Programme, known as 'Heartbeat Wales', is a UK national demonstration project. It is now part of the Health Promotion Authority for Wales. The purpose of the programme is to develop, mount, and evaluate a strategy that will reduce the prevalence of generally accepted risk factors for cardiovascular disease—with the long-term aim of contributing to a sustained reduction in coronary heart disease, morbidity, and mortality in the general population of Wales, particularly in those under the age of 65.

The evaluation of the project is as much concerned with the process of change as it is with the measure of outcome. The measurement of outcome indicators, and the attribution of cause and effect in community-based programmes pose special problems for evaluation. A quasi-experimental design is proposed for the Welsh Heart Programme which compares changes achieved between the different health authority areas internally in Wales, and externally with a reference area outside of Wales. The use of a range of evaluation techniques based on network analysis, dose–effect analysis, and the measurement of unobtrusive indicators of change will be used to support assertions about cause and effect. To assess changes in health indicators it will be necessary to carry out a series of independent cross-sectional surveys of a random sample of the population in each health authority. As well as the more traditionally accepted health risks such as smoking, physical activity, and raised blood pressure, examination of perceived health and locus of control will be monitored along with changes in the environment.

As a demonstration project special attention is given to process evaluation. All local projects and programmes which are funded with support from the centre will be based on specific and measurable objectives addressing feasibility and generalizability as well as other desired outcomes.

On a national basis there are plans to monitor the impact and acceptability of the programme among the general public with the purpose of providing early feedback on specific aspects of the programme and to modify future plans and development. In addition, through survey and follow-up, it is planned to monitor the impact of the programme on health and education professionals and other community opinion leaders with a view to identifying mechanisms for greater involvement and commitment on their part to the programme.

Further information on the proposed evaluation design, the goals, objectives, and targets, and theoretical and practical aspects of the programme's implementation are available through a series of Welsh Heart Programme publications detailed in the bibliography.

References

Blackburn, H. (1983). Research and demonstration projects in community cardiovascular disease prevention. *Journal of Public Health Policy* **4**, 4.

Blackburn, H., Luepker, R., and Kune, F. G. (1984). *The Minnesota health programme: a research and demonstration project in cardiovascular disease prevention*. In Mattarazzo, J. *et al. Behavioural Health*. J. Wiley & Sons, New York.

Farquhar, J. W. (1978). The community based model in lifestyle intervention trials. *American Journal of Epidemiology* **108**, 103–11.

Farquhar, J. W., Fortmann, S. P., and Wood, P. D. (1983). Community studies of cardiovascular disease prevention. In *Prevention of coronary heart disease: practical management of risk factors* (eds N. Kaplan and J. Stamler). W. B. Saunders and Co., Philadelphia.

Farquhar, J. W., Fortmann, S. P., and Maccoby, N. *et al.* (1984a). *The Stanford five city project: design and methods, Stanford Heart Disease Prevention Programme*. Stanford University, School of Medicine, Stanford.

Farquhar, J. W., Maccoby, N., and Solomon, D. S. (1984b). Community applications of behavioural medicine. In *Handbook of behavioural medicine* (ed. W. D. Gentry). Guildford Press, New York.

Jacobs, D. R., Luepker, R. V., and Mittelmark, M. *et al.* (1985). Community wide prevention strategies: evaluation design of the Minnesota heart health programme. *Journal of Chronic Diseases* **00**, 000.

Nutbeam, D. and Catford J. C. (1987). The Welsh Heart Programme Evaluation Strategy: Progress, Plans and Possibilities. *Health Promotion* **2**, (1), 5–18.

Puska, P., Nissinen, A., and Salonen, J. T. *et al.* (1985). The community based strategy to prevent coronary heart disease: conclusions from the ten years of the North Karelia project. *Annual Reviews of Public Health* **00**, 000.

Rogers, E. (1983). *Diffusion of innovations*. The Free Press, London.

Rose, G. A., Blackbury, H. and Gillum, R. F. (1982). *Cardiovascular survey methods*. World Health Organization, Geneva.

Welsh Heart Programme Directorate (1985a). *'Take Heart': a consultative document on the development of community-based heart health initiatives within Wales*. Heartbeat Report, Vol. 1. Welsh Heart Programme, Cardiff.

Welsh Heart Programme Directorate (1985b). *Protocol and questionnaire*. Heartbeat Report, Vol. 2. Welsh Heart Programme, Cardiff.

Welsh Heart Programme Directorate (1986a). *Welsh heart health survey 1985: clinical survey manual*. Heartbeat Report, Vol. 3. Welsh Heart Programme, Cardiff.

Welsh Heart Programme Directorate (1986b). *'Pulse of Wales', preliminary report of the Welsh heart health survey 1985*. Heartbeat Report, Vol. 4. Welsh Heart Programme, Cardiff.

World Health Organization (1982). *Prevention of coronary heart disease: report of a WHO expert committee*. Technical Report Series, Vol. 678. World Health Organization, Geneva.

World Health Organisation (1983). Proposal for the Multi-national Monitoring of trends and determinants in Cardio-vascular disease and protocol (MONICA), Geneva.

World Health Organization (1985). *Countrywide integrated programme for prevention of non-communicable diseases; guidelines for monitoring and evaluation*. WHO Regional Office for Europe, Copenhagen.

World Health Organization (1986). *Community prevention and control of cardio-vascular diseases: report of a WHO expert committee*. Technical Report, 732, World Health Organization, Geneva.

10

The behavioural risk factor surveys in the United States 1981–1983

GARY HOGELIN

In recent years the United States has increasingly focused on certain behaviours as critical determinants of health. That focus has created national health objectives, new state legislation to change health-related behaviour, and considerably more data collected to describe the health-related behaviours of American adults. Increasingly, Americans recognize that behaviour plays a critical role in developing 9 of the 10 leading causes of premature death (Table 10.1) (MMWR 1985). As behaviour has become increasingly recognized as a health determinant, so the means of collecting and analysing data about health-related behaviour has become more important.

Health-related behaviour data in the United States can be gathered from such seemingly obscure sources as the Department of Defense and the Department of Commerce. At least 8 of the 13 cabinet-level offices of the United States Government (Department of Defense, Department of Health and Human Services, Department of Transportation, Department of Commerce, Department of Education, Department of the Treasury, Department of Justice, and Department of Agriculture) routinely collect information to describe one or more American health habits. The data are collected from tax receipts, criminal justice systems, and a host of surveys. For obvious reasons surveys produce our best source of information. It is beyond the scope of this chapter to describe all the health surveys that have been conducted in recent years. Rather, this chapter will review some of the Centers for Disease Control's efforts to help official state health agencies collect behavioural risk factor data, highlight some of the analyses from those data, and to suggest some data-collection policies which become evident from the analyses.

The need for behavioural risk factor data at the state level was born out of new federally sponsored health promotion/disease prevention programmes for the states. Health promotion and disease prevention depend on individual behaviour to encourage a healthy style of living as a means to enhance an individual's overall well-being (health promotion) or changes in behaviour to prevent specific diseases from manifesting (disease prevention). As part of

Table 10.1 Years of life lost and associated behaviours by cause of death, 1983, United States of America

Cause of mortality	Years of life lost before age 65	Associated behaviours
Accidents and adverse effects	2 219 000	Alcohol misuse, firearm ownership, speeding, failure to wear seat belt, cigarette smoking
Malignant neoplasms	1 808 000	Cigarette smoking, diet, failure to use screening tests, alcohol misuse
Diseases of the heart	1 559 000	Cigarette smoking, diet (obesity), failure to follow hypertension treatment, sedentary life style
Suicides, homicides	1 218 000	Alcohol misuse, response to stress, firearm ownership
Chronic liver disease and cirrhosis	248 000	Alcohol misuse
Cerebrovascular disease	226 000	Failure to follow hypertension treatment, detection
Congenital anomalies	134 000	
Chronic obstructive pulmonary disease and allied conditions	123 000	Cigarette smoking
Diabetes mellitus	115 000	Diet (obesity)
Pneumonia and influenza	106 000	Failure to take influenza immunization
Ten leading causes (total)	7 756 000	
All causes (total)	9 170 000	

a federal assistance programme to the states, the Centers for Disease Control in 1981 began assisting state health departments to collect data enabling the states to estimate the prevalences of various behavioural risks in their adult populations. At that time only one or two states (of the 50 states) had such data. With the CDC's assistance, 28 states and the District of Columbia were able to conduct surveys of behavioural risk factors from 1981 to 1983; most were conducted in 1982.

Because the states needed an inexpensive, relatively simple method to gather risk-factor data, the CDC chose to use telephone interviews of randomly selected households much like a polling organization would. As part of its assistance, a standard questionnaire was developed using questions from previously conducted national surveys, such as supplements to the Annual Health Interview Survey and a hypertension survey sponsored by the National Heart, Lung, and Blood Institute. Only questions on exercise were developed at the CDC because no consistent set of questions on that topic existed. The basic philosophy behind the questionnaire was to concentrate on actual behaviours rather than on attitudes or knowledge. It was purposely kept very short, taking less than 10 minutes to complete, permitting the individual states to add questions of local interest without over-burdening the respondent. Because every state used the core questionnaire, data could be compared among the states.

The core questionnaire provided a few questions on the following predominant risk areas: cigarette smoking, physical activity, alcohol misuse (including drinking and driving), height/weight status (obesity), hypertension, stress, and seat belt use. The questionnaire included basic demographic data items as well as appropriate transitional wording. Other assistance included CDC on-site training in survey operations, sampling, and interviewing skills.

The sampling plan used in most states was a three-stage cluster design (Waksberg 1978). That sampling plan was chosen for its relative ease of administration and its efficiency. The sampling plan's efficiency is gained in the first stage by identifying working blocks of residential telephone numbers or, conversely, by eliminating non-residential blocks of telephone numbers from the sample. The second stage of the sample randomly generated the last two digits of the telephone number. The third stage involved identifying a single, randomly selected adult from within the household.

The interviews typically were conducted during evenings and weekends. In some states, health department personnel conducted the interviews; in others, students conducted the interviews; and in others, interviewers with survey research firms were used. Usually the interviewers were women. Health agency personnel supervised questionnaire editing and monitored the interviews and survey procedures. Training in these functions was provided by CDC staff.

Surveys in each state followed a given set of procedures for identifying eligible respondents and for ensuring that an adequate attempt was made to reach a respondent at each selected telephone number. Only supervisors could replace a number that could not be reached or where the respondent refused an interview. Each interviewer was periodically monitored during interviewing and verification or repeat calls were made on a portion of completed calls to monitor interviewer compliance with the protocol. Each interview took 8 to 10 minutes to complete. Considering callbacks, no answers, etc., two interviews generally could be completed per hour of the interviewer's time.

During 1982, after most of the 28 states had completed their surveys, it became apparent that national estimates could be derived by conducting a final survey composed of all 22 states that had not completed surveys or which had used a different questionnaire. That supplemental survey was completed and the results aggregated with the states' surveys to produce national estimates (Gentry *et al*. 1985).

The methods and questionnaire used to conduct the supplemental survey were the same as those used for the 28 states and the District of Columbia. With comparable data collection methods, the samples from the 30 risk factor surveys were combined and treated as a stratified probability sample of the United States. Because the combined sample is more a by-product rather than the primary product of the risk factor surveys, the 'design' of the combined sample is less than optimal (statistically) than if the expressed goal of the programme had been to produce national estimates.

Weights were applied to individual respondents of the combined sample to compensate for the following:

1. Approximately equal sample sizes among states of widely varying population.
2. Varying probability of selection from a household.
3. Varying numbers of telephone numbers assigned to a household.
4. Variable cluster sizes.
5. The age, race, and sex distribution of the population represented in the data.
6. The growth of the population between the 1980 census and the midpoint of the risk factor survey—July 1, 1982 (Gentry *et al*. 1985).

In the unweighted data, men and young adults were under-represented whereas persons aged 25 to 44 and women were over-represented (Table 10.2) (Gentry *et al*. 1985). These discrepancies in the sample's demographic distribution compared with the United States population result from the joint effects of differential telephone coverage and survey non-response. They are, however, corrected somewhat by the adjustment that brings the weighted distribution of the sample by age, race, and sex in each individual survey population in line with the 1980 census data (Gentry *et al*. 1985).

Although the survey contains 22,236 interviews, the design effect is substantial. In other words, the effective sample size for analytical purposes is substantially reduced. Also, the response rates varied considerably from state to state but averaged 74 per cent when computed by the technique of the Council of American Survey Research Organizations. We have no information on the characteristics of the non-respondents. The total sample from

Table 10.2 Age, sex, and race distributions, unweighted and weighted, combined BRF surveys 1981–1983

Age group	Whites		Non-whites		Total sample	
	Unweighted	Weighted	Unweighted	Weighted	Unweighted	Weighted
18–24	11.2	15.2	3.2	3.5	14.4	18.7
25–34	21.9	19.3	5.0	4.0	26.9	23.3
35–44	15.5	13.5	3.2	2.5	18.7	16.0
45–54	10.7	12.3	2.2	2.0	12.9	14.3
55–64	11.4	12.0	1.8	1.5	13.2	13.5
64+	12.0	12.8	2.0	1.5	14.0	14.3
Total	82.7	85.1	17.4	15.0	100.1	100.1
Sex						
Male	35.7	40.8	7.0	7.0	42.7	47.8
Female	46.9	44.4	10.4	7.9	57.3	52.3

which participants were randomly identified represents 93 per cent of all United States households; 7 per cent of eligible respondents were excluded by not having a telephone. Finally, the data represent only self-reported behaviours.

The overall prevalences of the risk behaviours are provided in Table 10.3. Understandably, behavioural data are quite variable depending on how the particular behaviour is defined. Each behaviour is defined in the Glossary.

Because the data set covers a wide range of health-related behaviours rather than one particular behaviour, the possible analyses of such data is extensive and beyond the scope of this chapter. This presentation will focus on three particular behaviours: cigarette smoking, seat belt non-use, and drinking and driving. Some analyses completed from the data are highlighted to illustrate how those data can best serve the health promotion–disease prevention efforts in the United States.

Table 10.3 1981–1983 Behavioural risk factor prevalence estimates

Behavioural risk factor	Prevalence*	95% confidence interval
Overweight	22.6	(21.8–25.5)
Sedentary life style	12.1	(11.1–12.9)
Uncontrolled hypertension	4.0	(3.4–4.6)
Cigarette smoking	31.5	(30.2–32.7)
Binge drinking	22.7	(21.5–23.9)
Heavier drinking	8.7	(7.9–9.4)
Drinking and driving	6.1	(5.4–6.9)
Seat belt non-use	75.9	(74.7–77.1)

* Percentage of adults, 18 and over, at risk (see glossary for definitions of 'at risk').

Cigarette smoking has probably been the most studied and documented American health behaviour. There is little this study's data could do to greatly further our understanding of cigarette smoking. However, the data do point out two issues of data collection policy which are worthy of mention: trends and subpopulation-specific estimates. An analysis of those issues was undertaken by Remington *et al*. (1985) at the Centers for Disease Control.

The decline in smoking prevalence in the United States began in the early 1960s and continues today (Department of Health and Human Services 1979). The overall decrease in cigarette smoking has been primarily a result of the marked decline in the proportion of adult male smokers: from 51 per cent in 1965 to 33 per cent in 1985 (Fig. 10.1). In contrast, the rate among women has decreased only slightly, from 33 per cent in 1965 to 28 per cent in

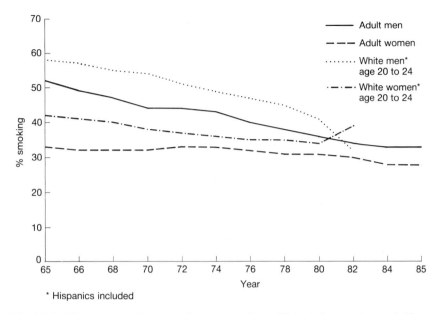

Fig. 10.1 Cigarette smoking trends among adults, United States, from 1965 to January–March 1985.

1985 (National Health Interview Survey 1985), and since 1978 there has been little change. Others have speculated that because of those relative shifts in the smoking rate among men and women, the rate of lung cancer in women will exceed the rate in men by the year 2000 (Starzyk 1983; Stolley 1983). If these trends continue, we may achieve 'equality' in the prevalences of smoking for men and women before 1990.

The greater decline in smoking among men can be attributed to higher rates of cessation and lower rates of starting among young men (Department of Health and Human Services 1983a). Among young whites (including Hispanics), the rate among men has continued to decline rapidly since 1965, whereas among young women, the gradual downward trend was offset by a substantial increase in 1982, with smoking rates comparable to the rate in 1965 (Fig. 10.1) (Department of Health and Human Services 1983b).

The rate of cigarette smoking among high school seniors peaked in the mid-1970s, decreased after that, but levelled off between 1980 and 1983 (Johnston *et al.* 1984). Despite these encouraging trends, individuals who smoked only occasionally in their senior year sharply increased their amount of smoking in the first year or two after high school (O'Malley *et al.* 1984). The behavioural risk factor surveys reveal that women between the age of 18 and 24 who graduated between 1976 and 1982 had the highest smoking rates. Other data similarly show that 17- to 18-year-old girls had a higher proportion of smokers than did 17- to 18-year-old boys (Department of Health and Human Services 1980). This may indicate that, for women, the decreasing trend of smoking at the time of high school graduation may be offset by an increase in the proportion of women who begin to smoke after graduation. The behavioural risk factor surveys reveal that women are not following the overall trend towards reduced smoking. In fact, the proportion of smokers among young white and Hispanic women of childbearing age appears to have increased. Those women represent a particularly important group to target for prevention and cessation programmes, before the well-known morbidity and mortality associated with smoking develops.

The human burden of motor vehicle collisions in the United States is extraordinary. In 1983, car and truck collisions resulted in nearly 30 000 occupant deaths (Cerelli 1984). Various studies have demonstrated that serious injuries and fatalities would decrease by at least 60 per cent if everyone used seat belts consistently (Robertson 1976; Campbell 1984).

Seat belt non-use varies in different geographic areas of the United States. The analysis of the geographic distinctions of seat belt non-use is provided by courtesy of Goldbaum and his colleagues, also of the Centers for Disease Control (Goldbaum *et al*. 19   ). Fig. 10.2 demonstrates the geographic variation in seat belt non-use in the US. Generally the western states reported

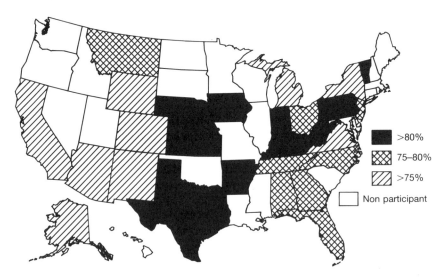

Fig. 10.2 Adjusted seat belt non-use by state (adjusted for sex, race–ethnicity, age, and education), behavioural risk factor surveys 1981–1983.

the lowest non-use rates. The geographic variation in that risk behaviour will become more evident in the near future. Increasing numbers of states are enacting mandatory seat belt use laws primarily as a result of federal pressure to enact such laws or face a national mandate for passive restraint systems in automobiles. As of this writing, 16 states have passed mandatory use laws (MMWR 1985). Although this map does not yet demonstrate the impact of laws on the prevalence on seat belt non-use, it does demonstrate that geographic distinctions in health behaviour do occur, and we can surmise that geographic distinctions will become more evident as the geographic distribution of health behaviours is influenced by legislation. In several Canadian provinces and New York state, seat belt non-use decreased by well over 50 per cent during the first few months that mandatory use laws were in effect (Table 10.4). Morbidity and mortality have been reported to decrease accordingly. Other geographic distinctions can be seen with overweight status and alcohol misuse—distinctions that may reflect cultural differences and demographic characteristics (Marks *et al*. 1985).

Table 10.4   Rates of seat belt non-use before and after mandatory use in Canadian Provinces and New York State

Province/State	Year law became effective	Percentage non-use before law	Percentage non-use after law
Ontario	1976	79	29*
British Columbia	1977	68	21*
Newfoundland	1982	84	23*
New York	1985	83	18†

* During first three months after law became effective.
† During first four months after law became effective (New York Behavioral Risk Factor Surveillance).

Alcohol is estimated to be involved in 58 per cent of fatal motor vehicle accidents (Conference on Alcohol, Drugs and Traffic Safety 1974). Recognition of the significant contribution of drunk driving to premature death and disability in the United States has led both government agencies and the private sector to make drunk driving a nationwide priority. The following analysis is by courtesy of Bradstock and her colleagues of the Centers for Disease Control (Bradstock *et al*. 1988).

As provided earlier (Table 10.3), 6.1 per cent of American adults admitted to drunk driving in the month preceding the interview. Significantly more men reported drinking and driving than women (9.2 per cent vs. 3.3 per cent), and the behaviour declines significantly with age. The youngest age category (18- to 24-year-olds) had the highest rates at 12.7 per cent (95 per cent CI = 10.0–15.9 per cent); and the lowest rates appeared among persons over the age of 65 and older (Table 10.5). Drinking and driving did not vary significantly by racial group. Seat belt use was negatively associated with drinking and driving (Table 10.6). Those who responded that they seldom or never use seat belts were more likely to report drinking and driving (7.4 per cent) than those who responded that they always or nearly always use seat belts (4.4 per cent) (RR = 1.6; 95 per cent CI = 1.2–2.2). That difference was significant for men but not for women; men who seldom or never use seat belts had rates of drinking and driving of 11.3 per cent versus 6.1 per cent of men who always or nearly always use seat belts (RR = 1.8, 95 per cent CI = 1.3–2.6). Cigarette smoking was strongly associated with drinking and driving. Heavy smokers (those who smoke more than one pack of cigarettes per day) were more than twice as likely to report driving after drinking than were non-smokers (11.3 per cent versus 4.7 per cent). Those who smoke one

Table 10.5 Drinking and driving by age, behavioural risk factors surveys, 1981–1983

Age in years	Rate			Rate ratio* total
	Male	Female	Total	
18–24	15.4%	9.9%	12.7%	1.00
25–44	11.6%	3.5%	7.5%	0.59
45–64	5.2%	0.9%	3.0%	0.23
65+	0.4%	0.0%	0.1%	0.01

* All differences statistically significant at the 0.05 level.

Table 10.6 Drinking and driving by seat belt usage, behavioural risk factor survey, 1981–1983

	Rate			Rate ratio* total
	Male	Female	Total	
Always/nearly always	6.1%	2.9%	4.4%	1.00
Seldom/never	11.3%	3.7%	7.4%	1.66

* Statistically significant at the 0.05 level.

pack per day or less had rates intermediate between heavy smokers and non-smokers.

Finally, the association between drinking and driving and an individual's behavioural response to stress was studied. Respondents were significantly more likely to drink and drive if they drink (21.0 per cent) or smoke (8.7 per cent) in response to stress than if they exercise (5.8 per cent) in response to stress. The behavioural risk factor surveys provided the states with baseline data. Aggregated, the surveys provided some insight into the associations between behaviour such as drinking and driving and other risk factors. Those associations between behaviours point to the synergistic effect those behaviours may have, each increasing the total risk to the individual. Drinking and driving accompanied by seat belt non-use is an obvious example of how the risk of injury or death is increased. The possibility of a health-risk clustering phenomenon has led some authors to call for reorganizing prevention efforts, going beyond the prevention of classical risk factors, such as drinking and smoking, to affect the common predisposing, enabling, and reinforcing factors that underlie the risk factors (Oullet *et al*. 1979). The rationale for trying to influence the factors underlying a particular behavioural risk is that unless the underlying behaviour is identified or prevented or treated, the behaviour will either recur or be replaced by others.

Conversely, the finding from the behavioural risk factor surveys, that both non-smokers and seat belt wearers are less likely to drink and drive, supports the notion that 'positive' behaviours may also cluster and be mutually reinforcing (Selzer *et al*. 1977). Although that issue needs more investigation, it certainly is a promising line of inquiry.

Discussion

We all ultimately seek to achieve reduced premature death and disability. Our approach to data collection and analysis can play a vital role in achieving that goal. For example, the analysis of cigarette smoking highlighted significant trends, particularly within certain sub-populations. As noted previously, the patterns of cigarette smoking varied in the four different groups. The analysis of trends was possible because the data was collected over a long time period, included a sufficiently large sample to permit sub-population estimates, and consistently relied on the same questions to determine the behaviour. Although those principles of periodic data collection sample size and consistency are familiar to us, we need only look beyond cigarette smoking to other behaviours to see how infrequently they are practiced in the United States. Trend analysis can be of value to those who are responsible for making public decisions by demonstrating that the trend is not following a gradual decline for all groups and is, in fact, increasing for some. The difference in trends may reflect various factors affecting smoking behaviour, such as directed advertising. To a public decision maker, trend analysis may point out where more direct models of intervention can be applied, such as school health education.

The analysis of seat belt non-use demonstrated a significant variation in the geographic distribution of this health-related behaviour. Moreover, Table 10.4 demonstrated that changes in the environment (in this instance through mandatory seat belt legislation) can play a decisive role in modifying an existing behavioural pattern. Similar but less dramatic changes can be shown in the effects of taxation and legal drinking age legislation on alcohol consumption and cigarette smoking. The geographic distinctions that arise or are modified by varying local laws and policies are clear evidence that the policymaker is making a difference.

The drinking and driving analysis also points to the value of integrated, comprehensive data. Those data demonstrate that health behaviours can and do cluster. The cluster effect can be demonstrated because the data were comprehensive—that is, information was collected on a number of health risk behaviours. The clustering phenomenon is critical to assessing total risk in the population as well as to a better understanding of the social context of the behaviours. To a public policymaker, the clustering phenomenon indicates that education programmes must be designed which can bring about behaviour change with respect to a broad range of health conditions. The phenomenon also means that educational programmes must prevent replacing one health risk behaviour with another and may prevent potentially harmful interaction between health behaviours.

For those intimately involved with collecting behavioural data, we must maintain a clear focus on the primary goal of reducing death and disability. We must maintain an awareness of how our data will help us achieve that goal. We must also actively use our data in the political arena. As the cost of traditional one-to-one intervention becomes increasingly prohibitive, broad societal and community-level changes instituted by public policymakers are our most cost-effective tools for encouraging positive changes in health behaviour. Reliable data will demonstrate to policymakers that health behaviours are amenable to action—they are influenced by social policies. Thus we can show public policymakers that their actions can make a difference. The behavioural risk factor surveys are new to the Centers for Disease Control and are new to those in the health promotion/disease prevention field. We are only beginning to understand how to collect and use the data effectively. We must look for ways to market our data to motivate policymakers to take action. In essence, we should look to our efforts in data collection as catalysts for the changes we seek.

Glossary: behavioural risk factor definitions

Overweight—At least 120 per cent of ideal weight (ideal weight defined as the mid-value of the medium-frame person on the 1959 Metropolitan Life Insurance height/weight tables).

Sedentary life style—Combined low level of activity from exercise, work, and recreation.

Uncontrolled hypertension—Person told by medical professionals that he/she was hypertensive and who still has high blood pressure.

Cigarette smoking—Current cigarette smoker.

Binge drinking—Person who has had five or more drinks on an occasion, one or more times in the past month.

Heavier drinking—Person whose average total alcoholic beverage intake exceeds 56 drinks a month.

Drinking and driving—Person who has driven after having too much to drink, one or more times in the past month.

Seat belt non-use—Person who states he/she uses seat belts only sometimes, seldom, or never while driving or riding in a car.

References

Bradstock, K., Marks, J., Forman, M. *et al*. (1988). Drinking and driving and health lifestyle in the United States: behavioural risk factor surveys. *Journal of Studies on Alcohol* **48**, (2), 147–52.

Campbell, B. (1984). *Safety belt injury reduction related to crash severity and front seated position*. HSRC Publication PR129. UNC Highway Safety Research Center, Chapel Hill, NC.

Cerelli, E. (1984). *The 1983 traffic fatalities early assessment*. DOT Publication No HS-806-5H. National Highway Traffic and Safety Administration, Washington, D.C.

Conference on Alcohol, Drugs and Traffic Safety (1974), Epidemiological issues about alcohol, other drugs, and highway safety. *Alcohol, drugs and traffic safety*. Proceedings of the Sixth International Conference on Alcohol, Drugs and Traffic Safety, Toronto.

Department of Health and Human Services (1979). *Smoking and health (PHS)*. Office of Smoking and Health, Rockville, MD.

Department of Health and Human Services (1980). *Promoting health, preventing disease*. National Institutes of Health, Washington, D.C.

Department of Health and Human Services (1983a). *The health consequences of smoking for women: a report for the Surgeon General*. Publication No. 410-889-1284. Office of Smoking and Health, Rockville, MD.

Department of Health and Human Services (1983b). *Health, United States*. Publication No. 84-1232. National Center for Health Statistics.

Gentry, E., Kalsbeek, W., Hogelin, G. *et al*. (1985). The behavioural risk factor surveys: design, methods and national estimates from combined state data. *Journal of Preventive Medicine* **1**, 9–14.

Goldbaum, G., Remington, P., Powell, K., *et al*. (1986). Seat belt nonuse in the United States: the behavioural risk factor surveys. *Journal of the American Medical Association* **18**, 2459–62.

Johnston, L., O'Malley, P., and Bachman, J. (1984). *Drugs and American high school students 1975–1983*. Department of Health and Human Services, No. 31–51. National Institute on Drug Abuse, Rockville, MD.

MMWR (1985). State legislature activities concerning the use of seat belts—United States.

Marks, J., Hogelin, G., and Gentry, E. (1985). State-specific prevalence estimates of behavioural risk factors. *Journal of Preventive Medicine* **1**, 1–8.

O'Malley, P., Bachman, J., and Johnston, L. (1984). Period, age and cohort effects on substance use among American youth. *American Journal of Public Health* **74**, 682–8.

Oullet, B., Rooneder, J., and Launch, J. (1979). Premature mortality attributable to smoking and hazardous drinking in Canada. *American Journal of Epidemiology* **109**, 451–63.

Remington, R. *et al*. (1985). Current smoking trends in the United States: the 1981–1983 behavioural risk factor surveys. *Journal of the American Medical Association* **253**, 2975–8.

Robertson, L. (1976). Estimates of motor vehicle seat belt effectiveness and use: implications for occupant crash protection. *American Journal of Public Health* **66**, 859–64.

Selzer, M. and Barton, E. (1977). The drunken driver: a psychological study. *Drug Alcohol Dependency* **2**, 239–53.

Starzyk, P. (1983). Lung cancer deaths: equality by 2000? *New England Journal of Medicine* **308**, 1289–90.

Stolley, P. (1983). Lung cancer in women: five years later, situation worse: *New England Journal of Medicine* **309**, 428–9.

Waksberg, J. (1978). Sampling methods for random digit dialing. *Journal of the American Statistical Association* **73**, 40–6.

11

National surveys of health behaviour in Finland

ESKO KALIMO

Introduction

This chapter is intended to provide a description and analysis of the research strategies which have led in Finland to the planning and implementation of a number of national large-scale surveys of varying aspects of health behaviour during the last 20 years. The emphasis is placed on the issues of research policy; the chapter aims at providing a background of the research issues in the studies and of the keen interest in public health oriented national surveys in the country since the mid 1960s. In addition, the use of the findings of the studies in planning and decision-making within the health system is briefly described. The chapter does not cover the substantive aspects of the findings of the surveys, but some of the prominent conceptual issues are touched in order to help to understand the development of the research policy in this area.

The chapter is divided into four main sections. The first section discusses the main trends of the research policy in national surveys of health behaviour, and it is followed by a section on the conceptual framework used in these studies. The third section provides more detailed information about the main national surveys of health behaviour. The chapter ends with conclusions, which cover also the recent developments in research policy for studies on health behaviour.

The national health policy during the last 20 years in Finland reflects the growing role of the society in the health system and an increasing interest in health promotion with the adoption of the leading ideas of the WHO policy for Health for All by the Year 2000, in which primary health care (PHC) is the priority issue in health policy. The value of equity in health and accessibility to health services has played a prominent role in planning and implementing national health policies in Finland during the last twenty years. Yet, these trends are not necessarily new; for example, the hospitals have mostly been jointly owned by the communities for the past 200 years and many preventive activities have been emphasized and implemented in growing numbers in a national scale during the last 100 years.

The above trends in health policy are not unique in Finland but the strength of the adherence to the healthy policy goals and the related possibilities of implementing the necessary measures may be a characteristic which differentiates the situation in Finland from some other countries. Accordingly, the orientation towards health-promotive activities in Finland has developed in the following way. One may characterize the last 20 years by noting a fresh interest in the prevention of common diseases in the country in the mid 1960s, which was followed by a widening interest in the prevention of disability to work and rehabilitation in the early 1970s. This developed in a few years into an interest in the issue of maintaining the ability to function and work, which in the late 1970s deepened into an interest in measures aiming at health promotion.

The above orientation towards health-promotive activities reflects the application of the same views about the 'welfare state' as in the goal of health for the WHO global strategy for the Health for All by the Year 2000 (WHO 1981), which emphasizes a socially and economically productive life and 'more life to years' and 'more health to life' (WHO 1985), that is, socially defined capacities of the individual with a strong orientation towards aspects of positive health.

Trends in research policy

In order to understand the formation of a research policy, it is useful to pay attention to the source of financial support to research. In Finland a specific characteristic of institutions in public health and social security administration is that most of them have research departments or research units of their own (Kalimo 1971). This means that planners and decision-makers in this area have research facilities at their disposal with which they can collaborate for the development of the health and health-related activities. The latter concept is here used in a broad sense, as suggested by the World Health Organization (WHO 1981), since this system in Finland comprises of many social insurance and social welfare institutions which fairly directly deal with the problems of the ill health of the people (Kaitaranta and Purola 1973). Since national surveys are usually expensive research projects, the resources for the national surveys covering also health behaviour in Finland have been available from those governmental or other public institutions who are involved in the administration of health or health-related activities.

Therefore, the Finnish research policy in studies on health behaviour reflects the trends in health policy and in the orientation towards preventive and health-promotive activities, as described in the preceding section.

This means that health behaviour has been the main focus only in the more recent national surveys conducted since the late 1970s. Nevertheless, the interest in primary health care, and prevention and health promotion in general, has been an important background motive in focusing the national surveys. Consequently many surveys, although their main emphasis has been on illness behaviour and sick-role behaviour, have included aspects of health behaviour. For this reason, several national surveys whose main objective has been related to health systems research or epidemiological research have been included in this paper.

The Finnish national surveys have accordingly had a practical purpose; they have been expected to provide information which would help the planners and decision-makers to solve a specific problem or to achieve a specific goal. The researchers have been aware of the expectations regarding the applicability—but not the content—of the findings and conclusions of the surveys. The planners and decision-makers have given sufficient freedom to the researchers. On the other hand, the latter have been expected to conduct the surveys in a scientifically acceptable way. The have been expected to provide scientifically valid findings rather than findings which would support politically suitable measures. This scientific freedom which irrespective of the financing of the surveys has been given to the researchers has made it possible to conduct the surveys in a way that meets the scientific criteria.

The selection of the survey technique, either by household interviews or mailed questionnaires, as the method of collecting the data has been based on the interest in learning about different characteristics of the same person, for assessing the inter-relationships at the level of an individual, since it has been seen by the researchers that the health of the individual citizens finally was the main object of the policy measures which they were expected to develop by the surveys. Correspondingly, also the information was mostly needed at the level of an individual, and besides many data were available only directly from the individuals by questioning them. The survey technique with multi-variate statistical techniques had been applied in the country already in the 1950s and this had provided the researchers with sufficient experience from the use of large-scale surveys.

The fairly adequate resources supporting the surveys included data-processing facilities for large data-sets. The interest of the decision-makers in national health problems and the available resources to support even large-scale studies inspired the researchers to draw nationally representative samples.

Conceptual aspects

The collection of large sets of empirical data was not seen as justified without developing adequate conceptual models which would help to decide on the necessary variables and guide the analysis of the data and the interpretation of the findings. Many of these concepts were taken from social science or behavioural research, since the object to be explained was either human behaviour or processes of social organizations. Since these concepts had to be applied to health issues, medical science expertise was also called for.

Most of the national surveys have been conducted by multi-disciplinary teams of researchers. The three basic aspects of health, as given already in the concept of health in the Constitution of the World Health Organization, were from the beginning seen as essential in surveys of health behaviour and related issues in Finland. The biological concept of health or well-being, the social concept of health or well-fare, and the psychological concept of health or well-feeling have each been understood to form a conceptually separate entity, which has its specific role in understanding the concept of health in general terms and which can also be approached separately by operational methods in surveys. In particular Purola (1972) has developed this conceptual reasoning, which seems to have explanatory power not only at the individual but also at the aggregate level. Related models have also been developed on sickness behaviour (Purola *et al.* 1973). In these models the concepts of predisposing and enabling factors affecting the illness behaviour, and especially the use of health services, can finally be traced back to the health belief model (Becker 1974) which was originally developed to explain health behaviour by Rosenstock (1974).

A specific characteristic of the conceptual models used is the application of the nomenclature to the issues of ill health. Experience suggests that not only at the conceptual level but also in empirical studies it is easier to deal with phenomena that describe ill health rather than good health. Although it may not be simple to transform the findings on ill health to apply also to the planning of measures promoting good health, serious attention needs to be paid to the possibilities of adapting the conceptual models developed in terms of ill-health, illness behaviour and sick-role behaviour to prevention of disease and disability and to health promotion.

Although most of these models have used social or behavioural science concepts, the models have been given in terms of systems theory, which probably has helped to communicate the meaning of the models to scholars from other disciplines.

Description of national surveys

National health and social security interview surveys

The idea for this series of consecutive national surveys was originated in 1963, when making preparations for the implementation of the national sickness insurance scheme in the following year. In order to evaluate the achievement of the health policy objectives of the scheme, it was then decided to carry out a two-phase survey in 1964 and 1968 to learn about the equity in health services use and families' direct costs of health care in relation to the health needs. The third survey was carried out along the same lines in 1976 and the fourth survey is in preparation for implementation in 1987. These surveys have been evaluative of the primary care oriented health policy in the country as well as of the measures used to achieve the objectives of the policy. The surveys were carried out by the Research Institute for Social Security of the Social Insurance Institution, of which the parent institute administers the national sickness insurance scheme. The National Board of Health within the Ministry of Social Affairs and Health collaborated in the field work of the surveys.

The main body of the data collected in these surveys covers people's illness behaviour and sick-role behaviour. The first phase of the survey was a pioneering nationwide health-systems research study in the country, and this made it necessary to prepare also conceptual models in this area. In addition to the main body of data, each survey has included a number of questions on health behaviour, for example use of physician services for preventive purposes, smoking, etc.

The data were collected in each phase of the survey by public health nurses using personal household interviews. In each phase about 7000 families and their 25 000 family members were interviewed. The sample was representative of the total non-institutionalized population of the country (Purola *et al*. 1968; Purola *et al*. 1974; Kalimo *et al*. 1982).

The second phase of the survey was carried out in 1968 at the same time as the International Collaborative Study of Medical Care Utilization (WHO/ICS-MCU) in Finland and in six other countries (Kohn and White 1976), which made it possible to compare the situation not only in the Finnish study area but throughout Finland with 11 study areas from other countries. Although the international survey was mostly on illness behaviour and sick-role behaviour, even this survey covered a number of aspects of health behaviour.

The mini-Finland health survey

The main purpose of this national survey was to obtain mainly epidemiological information which would help to develop health promotion, health care, and rehabilitation, as well as the health information system in the country. The origin of this survey was in the health examination surveys of the Social Insurance Institution, which were started in 1965, using a mobile clinic. The Mini-Finland Health Survey was conducted by the two research institutes of the SII, the Rehabilitation Research Centre and the Research Institute for Social Security, during 1977–1980.

The data which were collected in the health interview and the health examination parts of this survey as well as in subsequent, more detailed clinical examinations, cover not only a fairly comprehensive assessment of the health status of the persons but also a large number of potential risk factors in their behavioural and social environment. The purpose was to analyse the relationships between the indicators of health, risk factors, and other environmental factors and to draw conclusions to help to plan preventive and health-promotive activities. A fairly large number of indicators of health behaviour was included in this survey.

The survey covered a representative sample of those who were at least 30 years of age in the whole country. The sample was 8000 persons in 40 different areas of the country (Aromaa *et al*. 1985–6).

A large number of reports of specific issues have been prepared on this study, and the main English reports are in preparation.

A national questionnaire survey of sickness absenteeism from work

The reasons which led to this national questionnaire survey of sickness absenteeism from work and on the factors affecting it were in the growth of sickness absenteeism rates in many European countries in the early 1970s. The Research Institute for Social Security was therefore asked by the Social Insurance Institution to conduct a study on this highly topical issue in order to find out the sickness absenteeism rates in different occupational groups and to learn about the factors which contributed to it. In the background there was an interest to use the findings of the study to plan measures which would help to alleviate sickness absenteeism from work by strengthening preventive and health-promotive activities.

The questionnaire also covered various features in health behaviour in order to learn about the health culture of different occupational groups so that the behavioural aspects of sickness absenteeism could be placed in a broader perspective. Conceptually, this survey followed the models developed for the National Health and Social Security Interview Surveys.

The survey covered a sample of the salaried population in different occupational sectors, excluding the smallest work places. About 13 000 employees responded to the mailed questionnaire in 1974 (Nyman and Raitasalo 1978).

Although most of the data were related to the issue of sickness absenteeism, i.e. sick-role behaviour, increasing attention was paid to the use of the findings of the study to plan measures which would help to promote health-conducive life styles.

National questionnaire surveys of health behaviour

Towards the latter part of the 1970s there was a growing interest in the national health administration to have access to adequate data about people's health behaviour and the changes in it. This was due partly to a long-term interest in preventive activities, which had been reflected in an increasing number of studies since the early 1960s, and partly to a growing attention to the need to plan health-promotive measures.

These annual surveys were started in 1978 by the Public Health Institute in collaboration with the National Board of Health. The main purpose of this series of surveys is to monitor the health behaviour of people of working age, especially their smoking and nutrition. The survey also covers the use of alcohol, dental hygiene, physical activity, and traffic safety.

The data are collected annually by mailed questionnaires to a sample of about 5 000 persons. The results are published in simple tabular reports (e.g. Puska and Piha 1984) and in scientific reports on specific issues.

National interview surveys of health education

This national survey has been conducted by the Central Statistical Office at the request of the National Board of Health. The main objective of the survey is to obtain basic facts about timely problems in health behaviour for planning health education. The survey has been planned so that it can cover opinions, knowledge, and beliefs. The availability of the basic results, immediately after the field work, has been emphasized as well as the repetition of the survey at short intervals to make it possible to monitor changes in essential aspects of health behaviour.

Smoking has been the key issue of the survey but also nutritional issues, use of alcohol and related problems, abortions, small group activities to support health behaviour, obesity, perceived amount of health education, medicines, and traffic have been frequently monitored issues.

The survey has been conducted twice a year since 1979 on a nationwide sample of about 2000 persons in the age group of 15–64 years. In the first years most of the data were collected by telephone interviews, and later by personal interviews only (e.g. National Board of Health 1979).

National questionnaire surveys of occupational health care

The Occupational Health Act in Finland pre-supposes that every industrially active person in the working age group is covered by an occupational health service. The introduction of this act into force at the beginning of 1979 also reflected political support for preventive and health-promotive goals, since these were the main reasons for setting up a comprehensive occupational health service in the country with mainly preventive objectives.

Since public support for the occupational health services is directed through the sickness insurance scheme, the Social Insurance Institution asked its Research Institute for Social Security to conduct a national questionnaire survey of the adult working population in two phases. This survey was to follow up the changes in the coverage of the population by the occupational health services as well as in essential factors affecting their behaviour related to health and sickness and the perceived work-related health risks. By comparing the findings from the two studies, conducted in 1981 and 1985, it is expected to obtain evaluative information about the functional adequacy and effectiveness of the occupational health services for the further development of the occupational health policy in the country.

Most of the aspects of health behaviour covered in the survey are work related and due to the data collection method used—mailed questionnaires— reflect the perceived views of the individuals and their psycho-social working environment.

The first phase of the study covered small work places and construction work only, since in the other occupational sectors occupational health services had already been developed by that time in such large numbers that no 'before' survey was considered necessary (Karisto and Keinänen 1985; Raitasalo and Riska 1985). The data of the second phase have been collected by mailed questionnaires to employers, employees, and occupational health service units in about 1300 work places and to their 16 000 employees, which formed a representative sample of persons working in salaried occupations (Lehtonen and Raitasalo 1985).

Conclusions

It was seen that only two of the six national surveys described above were carried out primarily to assess health behaviour. These two surveys were also relatively recent and are repeated once or twice annually. They are supported by the National Board of Health and are meant to provide up-to-date findings about specific aspects of health behaviour.

The four other national surveys covered only some aspects of health behaviour, which was not a priority issue in the surveys. However, all these four surveys shared an interest in primary health care, prevention and health promotion, and therefore the findings of even these surveys have turned out to be useful in planning health-promotive activities.

These four national surveys also shared an interest in using fairly detailed conceptual frameworks, often with social science orientation, in applying multi-variate statistical techniques and in reporting the findings in lengthy main reports of the survey. The specific research orientation in these four national surveys can be further characterized as follows:

- The research design has been evaluative of the national health policy and/ or its specific activities.
- Health behaviour and health services have been conceived as an inter-related system, in which the viewpoint of a single individual has been emphasized—but as part of the social system which greatly determines his lifestyle.
- Consequently health and sickness have often been conceived as perceived entities, although their social and biological aspects have also been conceptually and empirically covered.

- The surveys have been carried out by multi-disciplinary teams which have brought behavioural and social science expertise into health research.
- Survey methodology either by personal interviews or mailed questionnaires has been used.
- Conceptual development has been considered necessary to guide the planning of the research design and the analysis of the data.
- The surveys have been financed by sources that also finance health and health-related activities, which has affected the setting of the research problems according to the interests of the decision-makers and, on the other hand, helped to apply the findings into health and social security planning, administration, and policy making.
- Although starting from a single object, the surveys have covered a fairly broad range of issues, since this has been expected to provide a better environment for the data to be interpreted.
- Collaboration has been sought with international organizations or international research teams to learn about cross-national differences and specific Finnish characteristics in people's health-related behaviour and the health system.

Nationally representative data about fairly large samples, allowing an analysis of differences by population group are available over a period of 20 years in Finland. It is evident, however, that more detailed data about health behaviour have been collected starting in the late 1970s and that, on the other hand, these studies lack a deeper conceptual orientation and a detailed statistical analysis, so that conclusions could be drawn about relationships among various aspects of health behaviour and about factors affecting them. Recently the need for successive monitoring of health behaviour has been emphasized so that data would be available to assess the outcome of specific activities of health education and other health promotive measures, as well as to suggest needs for new activities when changes in health habits take place.

These views were also held by the Advisory Committee for Health Education which emphasized in its general plan for the development of health education for 1984–8 that the objective of the monitoring of health behaviour should be that the development of the health behaviour of the adult population can be followed with sufficient validity and accuracy, and sufficiently often. The Advisory Committee suggested a follow-up interval of one year. It also stressed that the results be made available quickly and analysed by population groups. This monitoring should not only focus on health behaviour but also on specific prerequisites for changing it, e.g. knowledge, attitudes, social support, environmental factors, services, etc. It also held that the annual surveys be accompanied by larger evaluative studies, for instance at five year intervals, based on research of population samples in the field (National Board of Health 1983).

Right now the National Board of Health plans to support the monitoring of health behaviour in the country by strengthening the coordination of the research policy of the research institutes in this area and by enhancing appropriate collaboration among the related research activities and forthcoming national surveys of health behaviour.

Summary

National surveys of health behaviour in Finland

The purpose of the chapter is to describe and analyse the research strategies which have been used in Finland during the last twenty years in national large-scale surveys of health behaviour. The paper discusses the research interests behind the studies as well as the use of the findings in planning and decision making. The paper is on the research policy in this area in Finland and it does not cover the substantive findings of the surveys.

Since the early 1960s nationwide surveys have been conducted in Finland to provide information about essential issues of health, health care and health promotion in order to develop the national health policy and the measures following from it. The justification for the studies, making available the necessary resources for them, has been given either in terms of topical health policy issues or health problems brought under public discussion.

Another characteristic of the studies has been the close relationship between the national health and/or social security administration and the research activities. The studies have been action-oriented and the decision-makers have been involved in setting the objectives of the study as well as in the application of the results to health and social security policy making and related planning and administration in the Ministry of Social Affairs and Health, the Social Insurance Institution, as well as in other relevant institutions.

This close relationship between the decision-makers and researchers has helped to focus the studies on current issues, but simultaneously it has lessened the interest that has been paid to the issues of health promotion.

The chapter covers the following nationwide studies:

• National Health and Social Security Interview Surveys, which have been conducted by the Research Institute for Social Security of the Social Insurance Institution, Finland, in collaboration with the National Board of Health, in 1964, 1968, and 1976.
• The Mini-Finland Health Survey, which has been conducted by the Rehabilitation Research Centre and the Research Institute for Social Security of the Social Insurance Institution, Finland, in 1977–1980. This survey follows the tradition of the health examination surveys of the Social Insurance Institution, which were started in 1965, using a mobile clinic.

- A Nationwide Questionnaire Survey of Sickness Absenteeism from Work, which was conducted by the Research Institute for Social Security of the Social Insurance Institution, Finland, in 1974 on an issue which was highly topical at that time.
- National Questionnaire Surveys of Health Behaviour, which have been conducted by the Public Health Institute annually since 1978.
- National Interview Surveys of Health Education, which have been conducted by the National Board of Health twice annually since 1979.
- National Questionnaire Surveys of Occupational Health Care, which have been conducted by the Research Institute for Social Security of the Social Insurance Institution, Finland, in 1981 and in 1985.

All the nationwide surveys described in the chapter contain a number of indicators of health behaviour and other factors which are of interest from the viewpoint of health promotion. The reports have been focused partly on other issues, sometimes at the expense of analysing the variables which are the most relevant in view of applications to support health promotion. In spite of these other interests, the studies form a growing data base over 20 years, on which basis some aspects of the health behaviour of the Finnish population are now fairly well known, although more detailed data are needed on specific aspects of health behaviour and on their changes over time. The research activities are presently co-ordinated to strengthen the data base available from the national surveys in the future.

References

Aromaa, A. *et al.* (1985–6). *The execution of the mini-Finland health survey*, Parts 1– 4, English summaries. Social Insurance Institution, Finland, Helsinki and Turku.

Becker, M. H. (ed.) (1974). *The health belief model and personal health behaviour*. Slack, Thorofare, NJ.

Kaitaranta, H. and Purola, T. (1973). A systems-oriented approach to the consumption of medical commodities. *Social Science and Medicine* 7, 531–40.

Kalimo, E. (1971). Medical care research in the planning of social security in Finland. *Medical Care* 9, 304–310.

Kalimo, E. *et al.* (1982). *Need, use and expenses of health services in Finland 1964– 1976*. English summary. Social Insurance Institution, Finland, Helsinki.

Karisto, A. and Keinänen, T. (1985). *Working conditions in the construction industry and the need to develop occupational health care in the early 1980s*. English summary. Social Insurance Institution, Finland, Helsinki.

Kohn, R. and White, K. L. (eds) (1976). *Health care: an international study.* Oxford University Press, London.

Lehtonen, R. and Raitasalo, R. (1985). SII study of industrial health services. English summary. *Sosiaalivakuutus* 23, 262.

National Board of Health (1979). *Aikuisväestön terveyskasvatustutkimus I. Kevät 1979*. Lääkintöhallitus, Helsinki.

National Board of Health (1983). *General plan for the development of health education for 1984–88. Recommendation of the Advisory Committee for Health Education.* National Board of Health, Helsinki.

Nyman, K. and Raitasalo, R. (1978). *Työstä poissaolot ja niihin vaikuttavat tekijät Suomessa.* Social Insurance Institution, Finland, Helsinki.

Purola, T. (1972). A systems approach to health and health policy. *Medical Care* **10**, 373–9.

Purola, T. *et al.* (1968). *The utilization of the medical services and its relationship to morbidity, health resources and social factors.* Social Insurance Institution, Finland, Helsinki.

Purola, T. *et al.* (1973). National health insurance in Finland: its impact and evaluation. *International Journal of Health Services* **3**, 69–80.

Purola, T. *et al.* (1974). *Health services use and health status under national sickness insurance.* Social Insurance Institution, Finland, Helsinki.

Puska, P. and Piha, T. (1984). *Suomalaisen aikuisväestön terveyskäyttäytyminen. Kevät 1984.* Public Health Institute, Helsinki.

Raitasalo, R. and Riska, E. (1985). *Need for development of occupational health care at small places of work.* English summary. Social Insurance Institution, Finland, Helsinki.

Rosenstock, I. M. (1974). Historical origins of the health belief model. In *The health belief model and personal health behaviour* (ed. M. H. Becker), pp. 1–8. Slack, Thorofare, NJ.

WHO (1981). *Global strategy for health by all for the year 2000.* World Health Organization, Geneva.

WHO (1985). *Targets for health for all.* World Health Organization, Copenhagen.

SECTION D

Research on health behaviour in local environments

INTRODUCTION

Ilona Kickbusch

An approach most useful for planning health promotion action is to start from settings of everyday life—where people live, work, love, and play.

In this section several of these settings are introduced and discussed in their relevance to health promotion: the home and family setting, the influence of supportive environments on young people's health, the relevance of the workplace, and the community setting. The type of research presented here can give us clues how to understand health behaviours as patterned not only by individual traits but collective values and environmental impacts.

A research tool that needs to be further developed is the community health profile or community diagnosis. It could assist with the dialogue on health within the community, particularly if performed by or with strong support from members of the community themselves. Such data on local health cultures would facilitate discussions between all health participants in the community and open avenues to innovative approaches to community health promotion and planning at local level.

Stronger focus also needs to be placed on the communities' total health potential and its caring resource. Serious thought must be given to mechanisms that will promote solidarity and care within the community and which at the same time help to overcome the undue burden of caring responsibilities put on women.

Finally, a major challenge lies with developing a more in-depth understanding of the interaction between social and physical environments and the health of individuals and communities particularly in urban settings. Of importance are long-term stressors, chronicity of certain conditions, and a wide range of mental health problems.

The World Health Organization's 'Healthy Cities' project is an attempt to develop action in health promotion at local level. It will need to be supported by research that changes its focus in the directions indicated above and partly reflected in the chapters in this section.

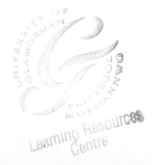

12

Health beliefs and behaviour in the home
ROISIN PILL

Introduction

The reader may be forgiven for finding the title distinctly ambiguous. Is the theme of this chapter research into health beliefs and behaviour that just happens to have been carried out in the home environment, or research that focuses on the home as the setting where families manage their health care? Both issues are addressed in this chapter. The first part uses my own work as an example of the former types of research, studies in which the home address is used as a convenient sampling unit for random population surveys or as a setting in which the respondents may be expected to talk more freely. Some of the problems, theoretical and methodological, facing anyone undertaking such a survey are illustrated and various strategies for dealing with them are offered. The second half examines the relatively scanty research data on how families actually function as a basic unit of health care, discusses the considerable gaps in our knowledge, and indicates possible future research initiatives.

Research on working-class mothers in South Wales

This research was carried out in collaboration with Dr. N. C. H. Stott and began with the aim of investigating the concept of individual responsibility for health and, in particular, the extent of people's awareness that day-to-day decisions regarding diet, exercise, habits, etc. were choices which influenced their future health. At that time, 1978, little had been published on health beliefs and behaviour and the paucity of research data in Britain was particularly noticeable (Stacey 1977; Illsley 1980). The aim was to develop measurements which could be replicated and thus be useful in assisting the choice of appropriate strategies for intervention and providing a tool for evaluating the success of health programmes.

The sample consisted of mothers with children under 16, the wives of skilled manual workers living with their husbands. This category was selected for two reasons. First, since women's attitudes and beliefs about illness had been demonstrated to influence both their own and their childrens' illness behaviour it was felt that their ideas about health and health maintenance were likely to be equally important for their families. Secondly, families of skilled manual workers (Registrar General Social Class IIIb) were chosen because they form a significant part of the total population of Britain and a majority of the population registered with the particular practice being used as a sample frame. The decision to approach these mothers in their homes was made on the grounds that they would feel more relaxed and talk more freely on their own territory.

The nature of the questions being addressed meant that interviewing was selected as the appropriate method. However, because of my past training as a social anthropologist and previous fieldwork experience, I was anxious not to use a standardized schedule. The decision was taken to conduct a pilot study (N = 41) to explore the language and the concepts used by the women in order to see whether it might be feasible to develop a tool for measuring the extent of awareness of the relevance of behavioural choices for life style (Pill and Stott 1982). The strategy followed relied heavily on Brown and Rutter's (1966) techniques for conducting interviews, with their emphasis on the elicitation of feelings and emotions. To this end the interviews were taped and transcribed, the tapes being used in order to aid coding and interpretation. In addition some standardized scales were administered, the health locus of control scales developed by Wallston *et al*. (1978), in order to compare these scores with my categorization (Pill and Stott 1981).

The main study was carried out on 204 mothers drawn from the same practice population but this time coming from semi-skilled and unskilled working class backgrounds (Registrar General Social Class IV and V). This group was selected because of the evidence that the lower socio-economic groups are most at risk in health matters, being less likely to take advantage of preventive services or carry out medically-approved practices (Townsend and Davidson 1982; Calnan 1985). The interviews were again done in the womens' homes by myself and two other interviewers. The larger sample size and the use of others necessitated a more structured schedule, detailed coding procedures, and analysis by computer. Despite the constraints imposed by a larger sample it was decided that it was important to utilize the insights offered by the pilot study and allow the interviewers to be more flexible in their questioning in certain sections of the interview, notably those dealing with attitudes to health, concepts of causation, and responsibility for health. The main aim was to test and validate the Index of Salience of Lifestyle (SLI)—the tool designed to measure the extent of awareness of the relevance of life style choices for health (Pill and Stott 1985a, 1987a). (This was based on a number of spontaneous references made to individual lifestyle in a set of five questions probing general beliefs about illness causation and prevention.) In order to provide some validation for this measure other beliefs and attitudes were explored, using a variety of techniques from open questions to standard scales. It was also decided to explore the relationship with measures of health behaviour, despite reservations about self-reported behaviour (Pill and Stott 1985b).

Two of the main problems I found doing these studies which are most relevant to this symposium were (*a*) the difficulties in eliciting concepts of *health* from the respondents, and (*b*) the operational definition and measurement of health behaviour.

Concepts of health

It was much easier in the pilot study, as it appears to have been in many of the studies purporting to be about health and health care, to get the mothers to talk about illness and illness behaviour rather than health. In fact I was able to demonstrate an association between readiness to recognize that individual behaviour (life style choices) had *some* part to play in illness causation and acceptance of the concept of individual responsibility, i.e. the notion that one was morally accountable for neglecting oneself and thereby reducing the level of resistance to illness. The difficulty may have been partly due to my own lack of confidence and uncertainty about how to elicit ideas about health as opposed to illness, and partly due to the fact that these are not very salient concepts for many of the women. Locker argues that the reason why accounts of health are usually less complex than accounts of illness is because a culture is likely to contain a more detailed and complex body of knowledge about those phenomena which present themselves as practical problems than it is about those which do not (Locker 1981, pp. 98–101). Being 'healthy' is not a status that has implications for action on the part of the individual or those around him; illness has to be managed whereas health can be taken for granted. Following this line of reasoning would imply that the health promotors would have to challenge this assumption and consider ways in which they could make the general public more convinced of the problematic status of being healthy. This may be difficult, as Baric (1969) has pointed out in his discussion of the 'at risk' role.

In the pilot study open questions such as 'what does being healthy mean to you?' 'would you think of yourself as basically a healthy person?' produced answers which were coded into three main categories. First, health as absence of illness, a concept also found by other researchers (Illsley 1980; Herzlich 1973); secondly, health as functional capacity, i.e. being able to cope with what one has to do; third, health as a positive condition of physical and mental well-being, expressed in terms such as 'being fresh and sort of bubbly, enthusiastic, and sort of cheerful'. There was evidence that mothers who were more aware of the role of life style factors in influencing health were more likely to have some positive concept of health and to view health as a dynamic relationship between the individual and her environment, susceptible to a variety of influences, some of which are under individual control (Stott and Pill 1980; Pill and Stott 1982).

An invitation to compare the health of this generation with their grand-parents also gave useful insights into the underlying factors they considered relevant to health. (This question was repeated on the main sample.) Here one third mentioned food, although this emphasis should not necessarily be construed as recognition of the role of individual choice because the availability of 'better' food or more food was seen as part of a general rise in the standard of living or changes in the modes of food production. After food, the factors most frequently mentioned were changes in prevalence of disease, perceived improvement in facilities and medical advances, followed by mention of changes in environmental and living conditions. Only 11 per cent thought people were healthier now because they were more aware of what they ought to be doing or because more information was available to help people to be healthy (Stott and Pill 1983). (The environmental issues also came out in discussions about illness prevention and causation.)

In the main study, in addition to some questions using a sentence-completion technique which produced rather stereotyped and not very useful answers, I attempted to get the mothers to talk about the factors they perceived as affecting their own health, and whether or not they felt they could do anything about them. To this end I adapted a technique developed in health education (Kreuter 1976). Having rated their own health by marking a line labelled at one end 'not at all healthy' and the other 'perfect health', they were asked 'what do you think is stopping you from being in perfect health?' The answers were classified as follows: one third recognized that life style choices were affecting their health, one half gave a particular condition or disease as the reason for not being in perfect health while 10 per cent talked about stress, tension, and worries affecting their health. The categories obviously overlapped but 42 per cent mentioned a condition or disease *only*, compared with 22 per cent who mentioned life style *only*. The women were also asked 'what do you feel you have in your favour?' and again only 30 per cent made any mention of life style choices under their own control, e.g. not smoking.

These findings support the original tentative hypothesis that a significant proportion of working class women do not appear to have a positive concept of health as something to be maintained. This technique seems to be quite acceptable and provides a quick way of exploring respondent attitudes which could be equally relevant for the clinician concerned to reinforce good practices and identify problem areas (Pill and Stott 1987b).

Problems with the definition and measurement of health behaviour

The concept of preventive health behaviour poses considerable problems for the researcher because of the lack of consistency in the concepts used, the operational definitions employed, and the different techniques used to collect data (see Anderson 1984). On theoretical grounds it seemed worth distinguishing between *procedures* (e.g. screening, immunizations, and check-ups) and *practices* (the day-to-day choices that have been defined by health professionals as having potential for maintaining health and preventing illness), and attempting to discover which factors most effectively discriminate between the two because they represent very different approaches to preventive behaviour. Procedures require professional involvement and compliance by the individual, whereas practices demand continual commitment from the individual with minimal involvement from health services. Furthermore, the health promotion lobby is increasingly concerned to empower the individual to integrate health practices into his or her day-to-day life.

In the main study the extent to which procedures and practices were interrelated in a sample and likely to be practised by the same people has been explored (Pill and Stott 1985b) and the findings do not support the idea of a general preventive orientation, and nor is there convincing support for the existence of hypothesized independent dimensions. Paradoxically our inability, along with that of other researchers, to explain more than about 20 per cent of the variance in self-reported behaviour* could be a source of inspiration for educators/professionals interested in health promotion. Preventive behaviour is obviously a complex area and it seems unlikely that any *single* variable, as yet unresearched, will reduce the level of unexplained variance substantially. It was argued (Pill and Stott 1985b) that this leaves about 80 per cent of the variance open to *situational* factors. The women's changing perceptions of their situation over time, opportunistic cues which trigger action, and the power of one-to-one continuing negotiation or practical demonstration have proved to be crucial in health behaviour changes (Stott 1983; Jordan-Marsh *et al.* 1983; Badura 1984).

Much more attention also needs to be paid to what behaviours people themselves perceive as relevant for health maintenance and claim actually to perform, regardless of their objective effectiveness or approval by the medical establishment. Following the pioneering work of Harris and Guten (1979) in the USA, I asked all the main sample respondents which three things they did to keep themselves healthy. What was interesting was that only 44 per cent named three things, suggesting again perhaps that the whole idea of positive health maintenance was not very familiar to them. Vague stereotyped answers were probed in an effort to ascertain exactly *what* a respondent meant/did (e.g. if she said she ate 'good food') and we also rated their replies on a five point scale according to the level of conviction they inspired (Pill and Stott 1986).

The behaviours mentioned were very similar to those described by Harris

---

* Using a combination of socio-demographic characteristics and various measures of beliefs and attitudes.

and Guten for their Cleveland sample and, more recently, by Calnan for a small British sample (Calnan 1986). Over three quarters reported some behaviour concerning nutrition, while just over half mentioned exercise, physical activity, or recreation, just over one in five mentioned rest, sleep, and relaxation. What can be seen as encouraging is the emphasis placed on personal health practices rather than procedures involving professionals. It was also found that women who named fewer health-protective behaviours scored significantly lower on the Index of Health Practices used in this study which was based on the classic research of the Alameda County Study (Berkman and Breslow 1983). On the other hand, some health promotors may find cause for concern in the significant proportion of this sample, admittedly the lowest socio-economic group, who appear to have little positive understanding or commitment to the notion of health maintenance.

The potential of the survey and other methodologies in the home environment

It is important to recognize that the traditional single-shot survey may well produce what Cornwell (1984) has called the 'public account', i.e. the answers deemed to be largely acceptable to others and therefore appropriate for producing in the artificial situation of the research interview. Such data are neither more nor less 'true' or 'valid' than data obtained in different ways or in different contexts. Their particular value lies in that they can be analysed to show what ideas or norms are perceived by various social categories or groups as essentially non-controversial and in conformity with the 'medical point of view'.

More than one interview with the same person will inevitably result in variation in what is said and how the respondent presents himself or herself. If we recognize that such variations are important data in their own right it becomes theoretically possible to exploit this by repeated interviews, thus giving an opportunity to analyse systematically the apparent contradictions and the ambivalence noted when only data from a single interview is available. As Hammersley and Atkinson (1983, p. 18) argue in a recent monograph on ethnography:

The fact that behaviour and attitude are often not stable across contexts and that the researcher may play an important part in shaping the context becomes central to the analysis. Indeed it is exploited for all it is worth. Data is not taken at face value but treated as a field of inference in which hypothetical patterns can be identified and then validity tested out.

Such issues as the use of non-verbal cues and the coding of feelings and emotional intensity of verbal statements following the tradition pioneered by Brown (Brown and Rutter 1966) could be profitably explored. Diaries have been used in health research but usually to provide data on symptoms or morbid episodes and utilization of services (Roughman and Haggerty 1972; Locker 1981; Alpert *et al*. 1969) and have been found to have drawbacks as data collection devices. A record of the day's activities may, however, have some potential as an aid to interviewing about health and health behaviours by giving the interviewer a chance to enquire about nutrition behaviours, use of leisure time, etc. (see Cullen and Phelps 1975; Cullen 1979).

Surveys can also be used to replicate the techniques described in the previous section, namely, the exploration of self-defined health behaviours and the invitation to respondents to talk about what barriers/facilitators they perceived as important to their present health. Less structured interviews, where the respondent is encouraged to tell his own story, can be analysed for their underlying logic in order to see whether certain concepts are given greater prominence by some groups than others (see Williams 1983). It may be, as Locker (1981) argues, that accounts of health are usually less complex than accounts of illness but more evidence is needed to test this proposition.

Given the practical difficulties of observing naturally occurring interactions in the home setting where health matters are spontaneously discussed, an alternative approach to the one-to-one research interview is the deliberate creation of a small group. Having initiated the discussion, the researchers can then observe and record the outcome. Focus groups are a qualitative data collection method adapted from market research, in which participants are brought together in small groups to discuss a topic of mutual interest. A recent example of this approach was a study by two social psychologists who showed several ways in which social interaction influences the formation of an individual's health belief schema for heart attacks (Morgan and Spanish 1985). In the home context this technique could be tried with a woman and two or three of the most significant members of her network, either friends or relatives. For example, it could be used to explore what knowledge was invoked in the discussion and to what extent exposure to the evaluations of other, in the form of either agreements or disagreements, produced modifications.

Husband and wife dyads are another possibility, partly to counter the almost exclusive reliance of the wife/mother's perspective and partly to obtain greater insight into the dynamics of family interaction and explore the implications for health behaviour. For example, my own research showed that several of the women mentioned that it was their husbands who were much keener on keeping fit, watching their weight, etc. than they themselves claimed to be and it was those views which influenced the pattern of family activities. Measures of the extent of agreement or disagreement between the partners about the importance of health maintenance obtained by joint interviewing could usefully complement data obtained separately.

This approach has potential for exploring the way that family health is organized, the priorities adopted and the way women act as buffers, maintaining the health of others by absorbing shortages themselves and allocating their resources of time and energy among their family. Graham (1985) has recently pointed out that this is precisely the area social scientists need to analyse if they are to increase understanding of the processes that govern health within the home. This leads us naturally on to consider what empirical research has been carried out in this area.

Research on the family as the basic unit of health care

When reviewing the literature on health care and the family Litman and Venters (1979) concluded that 'although interest in the role of the family in health and illness has increased greatly since the 1940s empirical enquiry has remained relatively limited, plagued by methodological imprecision and minimal integration with family theory'. There has been little advance in the past seven years. The reliance on the cross-sectional survey has meant that we have, as yet, little understanding of how families actually function as a basic unit of interaction and transaction in health care. This theme can be illustrated by three theoretical promising areas which appear to need further investigation:

1. The implications of the family life cycle for health beliefs and behaviour.
2. The issue of the transmission of health beliefs within the family.
3. The effect of the family's wider social links on its health beliefs and behaviour.

The concept of the life cycle has not been fully exploited; cross-sectional studies done at various stages of family development can identify some of the ways individuals define health and seek to maintain it, but longitudinal studies are also needed to explore such issues as the stability of beliefs over time, the impact of changing circumstances on both beliefs and reported behaviours, and to test more rigorously some of the hypotheses about the nature of the relationship between the two. There is a strong case for studies incorporating a time dimension into critical stages of the family life style, e.g. before and after marriage, before and after the first child, before and after retirement. An alternative research design that avoids some of the organizational and financial costs involved in a longitudinal approach is the use of intergenerational analysis (Litman 1971).

It is always assumed that the family plays a vital part in generating and reinforcing health beliefs and knowledge as part of the primary socialization process. However, the available empirical data suggests that the mechanism for transmission may not be as straightforward as had been thought. In an early survey looking at the influence of mothers on their childrens' health attitudes and behaviours, Mechanic (1964) concluded that maternal influence could not be regarded as particularly important but the sex and age status of the child were, and hypothesized that this finding revealed the importance of culturally-normative patterns inculcated by siblings, peers, teachers, etc. as well as the mother. Blaxter and Paterson (1982) examined the extent to which health attitudes, knowledge, and beliefs are passed from one generation of Aberdonian women to another and concluded that:

whether the analysis is of beliefs and values in general, or of the actual action taken during the survey period and the reasons given for that action, the *direct* familial link appeared to be weak (p. 185).

These findings suggest that more attention needs to be paid to the way that the family interacts with the wider community and the nature of the networks family members have (Chrisman 1977, pp. 363–367). At the individual level there is increasing recognition of the role of social networks in the understanding of illness behaviour (McKinlay 1981) and there is increasing evidence for their usefulness in understanding both the uptake of preventive procedures (Moody and Gray 1972) and the performance of personal health practices (Berkman and Syme 1979; Langlie 1977; Gottlieb and Green 1984; Dean 1986).

The only study I have come across which attempts to examine the way in which the family structure affects the health of its members, and the way in which health care is organized within the family is a study of 273 New Jersey families carried out by Pratt (1976). Mothers, fathers, and children were interviewed and indices of family functioning were developed, such as the level of conflict between husband and wife, extent and variety of interaction among family members, and the amount of autonomy accorded to children. Family links with the wider community were also examined. The dependent variables considered were performance of personal health practices, use of professional services, and level of health. Although one might criticize the operational definitions and the construction of the indices used, this study nevertheless represents an attempt to incorporate theory and explore specific propositions, and is written in such a way as to allow the reader to consider alternative hypotheses.

Several of her findings are particularly relevant to the symposium and deserve replication and further investigation. For example, it was found that:

1. The performance of good health practices by both women and children was significantly and positively associated with all types of extra-familial participation in the community.
2. The extent of the man's interaction in the family was particularly important for the woman's own health practices.

Conclusion

It will be apparent from the above that this field is a complex and demanding one—as yet largely virgin territory and offering considerable scope for imaginative exploratory research by those prepared to challenge preconceptions and be eclectic in their choice of research techniques. Apart from their academic interest such research can be of considerable relevance to those seeking to promote health, provided they attempt to understand the theoretical and methodological problems facing the researcher and, more especially, the implications of the way he or she chooses to resolve these problems.

In my view large-scale survey data on beliefs and behaviour collected in a research interview has value to health promoters because such data indicate the range and nature of the concepts and behaviours people feel are appropriate and generally acceptable. In-depth interviews, on the other hand, may indicate areas of ambivalence and ambiguity and reveal how people seek to make sense of their experience by invoking different bits of knowledge under different circumstances. The complexity of the relationship between expressed beliefs and attitudes and actual behaviour has been amply demonstrated in the work so far. It is clear that we are just beginning to explore the implications of the patterns of interaction both *within* the family and *between* the family and the wider society for the health behaviour of its members. It is as important for those seeking to promote health to be aware of the background variations in attitude, belief and behaviour among the various groups in their society/community as it is for them to appreciate that such variations are *not* static but constantly being modified and affirmed through interaction with others.

One of the main reasons for initiating the research that Dr. Stott and I have carried out in South Wales was to provide a properly-grounded theoretical and methodological base for health promotion and prevention in the context of primary care, so it is perhaps appropriate to end with a few words on this topic. It is frequently claimed that primary care health workers can be in a key position to promote health, and certainly it is agreed that one-to-one contacts, rather than mass campaigns, are probably the most effective way of bringing about changes in behaviour. Increasingly the emphasis is laid on the need to be 'patient centred' (Balint 1957; Byrne and Long 1976; Stott 1983; Pendleton *et al*. 1984). In this context it means being prepared to negotiate with the patient as an active partner in the promotion of his own health rather than attempting to impose professional views in an authoritarian way on a passive client (Katon and Kleinman 1981; Tuckett *et al*. 1985).

Awareness of the beliefs and knowledge held by the subgroups forming his clientele is essential for the health professional but can become a trap if this knowledge is used to stereotype clients (see Blalock and Devellis 1986; Pill and Stott 1987b) instead of being used on a basis for sensitive negotiation. Just as the researcher can develop a relationship with a respondent over time, obtaining different kinds of information and possibly allowing the informant an opportunity to construct and reconstruct his past experiences so, over time, the health professional can elicit the patient's ideas and practices, clarify discrepancies between his views and those of the patient, and try to move towards a mutually-acceptable agenda.

Such an approach is compatible with the philosophy underlying WHO policy on health promotion which stress that interventions should 'empower' the individual and not simply seek to impose officially-approved patterns of behaviour. The task facing health care professionals who hold a positive view about health promotion is to accept that people have a right to reject their advice while still remaining sufficiently professional and sensitive to react appropriately if a change of heart occurs in the patient.

Acknowledgements

The work described here was undertaken as part of a study of the health beliefs, attitudes, and behaviours of working class mothers granted to N.C.H. Stott by the Health Education Council. We would also like to acknowledge the help of the participants and the goodwill of our colleagues at the Department of General Practice, University of Wales College of Medicine.

References

Alpert, J. J., Kosa, J., and Haggerty, R. J. (1969). A month of illness and health care among low income families. *Public Health Reports* **82**, 705.

Anderson, R. (1984). *Health promotion: an overview*. European Monographs in Health Education Research, No. 6, pp. 1–76. Scottish Health Education Group, Edinburgh.

Badura, B. (1984). Lifestyle and health: some remarks on different view points. *Social Science and Medicine* **19**, 341–7.

Balint, M. (1957). *The doctor, his patient and the illness*. Tavistock, London.

Baric, L. (1969). Recognition of the 'at-risk' role: a means to influence health behaviour. *International Journal of Health Education* **12**, 24–34.

Berkman, L. and Breslow, L. (1983). *Health and ways of living*. Oxford University Press.

Berkman, L. F. and Syme, S. L. (1979). Social networks, host resistance and mortality: a nine-year follow-up study of Alameda county residents. *American Journal of Epidemiology* **109**, 186–204.

Blalock, G. J. and Devellis, B. McEvoy (1986). Stereotyping: the link between theory and practice. *Patient Education and Counselling* **8**, 17–25.

Blaxter, M. and Paterson, E. (1982). *Mothers and daughters: a three generational study of health attitudes and behaviour*. Heinemann, London.

Brown, G. W. and Rutter, M. (1966). The measurement of family activities and relationships. *Human Relations* **19**, 241–63.

Byrne, P. S. and Long, B. E. (1976). *Doctors talking to patients*. HMSO, London.

Calnan, M. (1985). Patterns in preventive behaviour: a study of women in middle age. *Social Science and Medicine* **20**, 263–8.

Calnan, M. (1986). Maintaining health and preventing illness: a comparison of the perceptions of women from different social classes. *Health Promotion* **1**, 167–78.

Chrisman, N. J. (1977). The health seeking process: an approach to the natural history of illness. *Culture, Medicine and Psychiatry* **1**, 351–78.

Cornwell, J. (1984). *Hard earned lives*. Tavistock, London.

Cullen, I. (1979). Urban social policy and the problem of family life; the use of an extended diary method to inform decision analysis. In *The sociology of the family* (ed. C. Harris). Sociological Review Monograph 28. University of Keele.

Cullen, I. and Phelps, E. (1975). *Diary Techniques and the Problem of Family Life*. Joint Unit for Planned Research, University College London.

Dean, K. (1986). 'Social support and health: pathways of influence. *Health Promotion* **1**, 133–50.

Gottlieb, N. H. and Green, L. W. (1984). Life events, social network, lifestyle and health: an analysis of the 1979 national survey of personal health practices and consequences. *Health Education Quarterly* **11**, 91–105.

Graham, H. (1985). Providers, negotiators and mediators: women as the hidden carers. In *Women, health and healing* (eds E. Lewin and V. Olesen). Tavistock, London.

Hammersley, M. and Atkinson, P. (1983). *Ethnography: principles in practice*. Tavistock, London.

Harris, D. M. and Guten, S. (1979). Health-protective behaviour: an exploratory study. *Journal of Health and Social Behaviour* **20**, 17–29.

Herzlich, C. (1973). *Health and illness*. Academic Press, London.

Illsley, R. (1980). *Professional or public health? Sociology in health and medicine*. Nuffield Trust, London.

Jordan-Marsh, M. A., Gilbert, J., Ford, J. D., and Kleeman, C. (1983). Lifestyle intervention: a conceptual framework. *Patient Education and Counselling* **6**, 29–38.

Katon, W. and Kleinman, A. (1981). Doctor–patient negotiation and other social science strategies in patient care. In *The relevance of social science for medicine* (eds L. Eisenberg and A. Kleinman), Chapter 12. Reidel, London.

Kreuter, M. W. (1976). An interaction model to facilitate health awareness and behaviour change. *Journal of School Health* **46**, 543–5.

Langlie, J. K. (1977). Social networks, health beliefs and preventive health behaviour. *Journal of Health and Social Behaviour* **18**, 244–60.

Litman, T. J. (1971). Health care and the family: a three generational analysis. *Medical Care* **9**, 67–81.

Litman, T. J. and Venters, M. (1979). Research on health care and the family: a methodological overview. *Social Science and Medicine* **13a**, 379–85.

Locker, D. (1981). *Symptoms and illness: the cognitive organisation of disorder*. Tavistock, London.

McKinlay, J. B. (1981). Social network influences on morbid episodes and the career of help seeking. In *The relevance of social science for medicine* (eds L. Eisenberg and A. Kleinman), Chapter 4. Reidel, London.

Mechanic, D. (1964). The influence of mothers on their children's health attitudes and behaviour. *Paediatrics* **33**, 444–53.

Moody, P. and Gray, R. (1972). Social class, social integration and the use of preventive health services. In *Patients, physicians and illness* (ed. E. G. Jaco). Free Press, New York.

Morgan, D. L. and Spanish, M. T. (1985). Social interaction and the cognitive organisation of health-relevant knowledge. *Sociology of Health and Illness* **7**, 401–21.

Pendleton, D., Schofield, T., Tate, P., and Havelock, P. (1984). *The consultation, an approach to learning and teaching*. Oxford University Press.

Pill, R. and Stott, N. C. H. (1981). Relationships between health locus of control and belief in the relevance of lifestyle to health. *Patient Counselling and Health Education* **3**, 95–9.

Pill, R. and Stott, N. C. H. (1982). Concepts of illness causation and responsibility: some preliminary data from a sample of working class mothers. *Social Science and Medicine* **16**, 43–52.

Pill, R. and Stott, N. C. H. (1985a). Choice or chance: further evidence on ideas of illness and responsibility for health. *Social Science and Medicine* **20**, 981–91.

Pill, R. and Stott, N. C. H. (1985b). Preventive procedures and practices among working class women: new data and fresh insights. *Social Science and Medicine* **21**, 975–83.

Pill, R. and Stott, N. C. H. (1986). Looking after themselves: health protective behaviour among British working class women. *Health Education Research* **1**, 111–19.

Pill, R. and Stott, N. C. H. (1987a). Development of a measure of potential health behaviour: a salience of lifestyle index. *Social Science and Medicine* **24**, 125–34.

Pill, R. and Stott, N. C. H. (1987b). The stereotype of 'working-class fatalism' and the challenge for primary care health promotion. *Health Education Research* **2**, 105–14.

Pratt, L. (1976). *Family structure and effective health behaviour*. Houghton Mifflin, Boston.

Roughman, K. and Haggerty, R. J. (1972). The diary as a research instrument in the study of health and illness behaviour experiences with a random sample of young families. *Medical Care* **10**, 143.

Stacey, M. (1977). Concepts of health and illness: a working paper on the concepts and their relevance for research. In *Health and healthy policy: priorities for research*. Report of an advisory panel to the Research Initiatives Board. Social Science Research Council, London.

Stott, N. C. H. (1983). *Primary health care: bridging the gap between theory and practice*. Springer Verlag, New York.

Stott, N. C. H. and Pill, R. (1980). *Health beliefs in an urban community*. Report to the DHSS, Department of General Practice, Welsh National School of Medicine.

Stott, N. C. H. and Pill, R. (1983). *A study of health beliefs, attitudes and behaviour among working class mothers*. Report to the Health Education Council, Department of General Practice, Welsh National School of Medicine.

Townsend, P. and Davidson, N. (eds) (1982). *Inequalities in health* (The Black Report). Penguin, London.

Tuckett, D., Boulton, M., Olsen, C., and Williams, A. (1985). *Meetings between experts: an approach to sharing ideas in medical consultations*. Tavistock, London.

Wallston, K., Wallston, B. and Devellis, R. (1978). Development of the multi-dimensional health locus of control (M.H.L.C.) scales. *Health Education Monograph* **3**, 160–9.

WHO Regional Office for Europe (1984). *Health promotion: a discussion document on the concept and principles*.

Williams, R. G. A. (1983). Concepts of health: an analysis of lay logic. *Sociology* **17**, 185–205.

13

The evolution of the juvenile health habit study 1977–1985

MATTI RIMPELÄ, ARJA RIMPELÄ, OSSI RAHKONEN, and
JUHA TEPERI

Introduction

The issue of smoking in young people has been widely debated for many years. In the 1950s the findings of epidemiological research added a new flavour to the debate and health interests became the main arguments in attempts to prevent young people from smoking (Rimpela 1978).

In Finland, an increasing trend in smoking among school children was one of the main motives behind the implementation of a nationwide smoking control policy in the middle of the 1970s (Leppo 1978; Leppo and Vertio 1986). No valid data on changes in young people's smoking were available. However, from numerous local surveys it was possible to demonstrate that, whereas smoking in boys had been established as a common habit by the late nineteenth century, the incidence of smoking in girls was ever increasing (Rimpela 1980). When the Tobacco Act was approved, one of the first measures was to plan an information system to evaluate the effect of anti-smoking activities.

In 1976 the National Board of Health decided to finance a study programme consisting of four consecutive nationwide surveys in 1977 and 1979. The first survey was carried out in February 1977, just before the implementation of the new act. The design of the study combined a trend survey and a panel study (Table 13.1). The data were collected by mailed questionnaires from samples of 3000 to 4000 adolescents. The findings of the surveys were encouraging. Response rate increased to 85 per cent. More than 70 per cent of the young people replied to all four panel questionnaires (Rimpela 1980). The National Board of Health has given continuous support to the surveys, which have been repeated biannually since 1979. The Juvenile Health Habit Study has become an integral part of the routine information system in health promotion.

Looking back over the ten years since the first survey, the evolution of the study has given us a lot to think about. The starting point was a need for information about changes in young people's smoking. From the beginning

Table 13.1 Design of the juvenile health habit study

Age	1977 Feb.	Sept.	1979 Feb.	Sept.	1981 Feb.	1983 Feb.	1985 Feb.	(1987...) Feb.
12	X		X		X	X	X	
		F						
14	X		FX		FX	FX	FX	
		F		F				
16	X		FX		FX	FX	FX	
		F		F				
18	X		FX		FX	FX	FX	
		F		F				
(20)			F					

(X = new sample for the follow-up of trends, F = panel study)

we had vague ideas about the life style approach (Rimpela and Eskola 1977), and questions dealing with other habits were added to the smoking questionnaire. Very soon we learned that the richness of our study design was the combination of a fixed core questionnaire and a more experimental part, which gave us an opportunity to test new ideas every second year. The focus of the survey has moved from smoking to the aggregation of health habits, perceived health, maturation, and social relations. Our impression is that the best way to develop new ideas is to analyse thoroughly what was done in the past and why it was done. In the light of the experience gained over the past ten years, we have reconstructed the evolution of the Juvenile Health Habit Study. The findings of this exercise are reported below.

From repressed to dominant structural interest

Robert Alford (1975) introduced a concept of a structural interest in the analysis of developments in health policy:

These interests are more than potential interest groups which are mainly waiting for an opportunity or the necessity of organizing to present demands or grievances to the appropriate authorities. Rather, structural interests either do not have to be organized in order to have their interests served or cannot be organized without a great difficulty.

Alford defined three categories of structural interests: dominant, challenging, and repressed. The structure and content of the existing health information systems tell us what are the dominant structural interests in our health policy. The information from routine sources ensure that those interests have automatically a central role to play in training, and evaluation, as well as in official reports and documents.

Before the era of the Tobacco Act the interests in the collection of information about smoking were in the category of repressed interests. There were no resources available and hardly any data on smoking was printed in public documents. According to Alford

... the nature of institutions guarantees that they [the repressed structural interests] will not be served unless extraordinary political energies are mobilized.

The approval of the Tobacco Act was the result of extraordinary political energies, and moved health interest related to smoking from the category of repressed interest into the category of dominant interest. Suddenly plenty of resources were available and the way to public reports was opened. Although our study programme primarily served the needs for smoking-specific information, it was possible to collect data on other health habits as well. This demonstrates well the nature of a challenging interest: it is served when it fits into the formula of a dominant one.

From the policy point of view a particular survey and an information system are in a different position. Single studies may have a limited scope without having any great impact on action. But when one of those studies becomes a part of routine administrative information, its framework is legitimized by national health authorities. During the first years we did not notice our role as servants of dominant structural interests. The conceptual considerations were carried out within the framework we had learned both in an academic department of public health and in planning for a nationwide smoking control programme. As Alford has put it 'People come to accept as inevitable what exists and even believe that it is right'. On the other hand, when dealing with the problems of young people and having the possibility to play with new items we became, step by step, increasingly aware of the gap between our approach and the information about health which is relevant to young people themselves.

At the outset we unquestioningly took the combination of administrative need for information and the epidemiological school of thought and planned our work accordingly. As a result, what is obvious to most people who are working with young people became obvious to us only after ten years of 'scientific' work. Whereas we had considered ourselves to be carrying out a study serving repressed and challenging interests, we gradually discovered we were merely serving the dominant structural interests of the Finnish health policy. This chapter describes the steps to this unfortunate discovery.

The conceptual frame of the study

As mentioned above, the patron of this study was the National Board of Health which needed information in order to evaluate the impact of its activities on smoking habits in young people. Starting from a smoking survey the aim was to develop a nationwide information system to follow up the changes in health habits. There existed two major administrative constraints. First, there was the need to establish representative information on changes in the whole population. Secondly, the study needed to pay particular attention to those age groups in which the risk of starting to smoke is high (young people aged 12 to 18 years). When taking into account the demand for representative data and the population density of Finland, the only suitable data collection method was a mailed questionnaire. The survey was devised in an academic department of public health. At that time we were very keen to apply epidemiological study designs and data analysis methods to the studies on health habits. We thought that the methodology as such was value-free. When the epidemiological approach was successful in the research on determinants of and changes in coronary heart diseases, it had been a useful tool in studies on the formation of and changes in a habit. Our aims were to:

- map changes in smoking behaviours over time by age, sex, place of residence, parent's social class, etc. (biannual surveys).
- describe the natural history of the smoking habit (a panel study),
- find out the specific determinants (risk factors) of smoking in young people (a panel study),
- explore the role of young people's own smoking habits as a determinant of their respiratory symptoms (a panel study).

The combination of a panel design and a trend study approach was made possible by the excellent population registry of Finland. Our sample consisted of all boys and girls born in defined days of July. Even after two years all boys and girls from the original cohort, and their new addresses, were easily picked up from the computerized population registry.

In retrospect it is easy to see the influence of the epidemiological tradition on our thinking. Habits were understood to be similar to diseases having a measurable point of starting and stopping. We were most interested in those habits which were labelled as risk factors, or at least as candidate risk factors, of major diseases: smoking, use of alcohol, consumption of animal fats, physical inactivity, poor dental hygiene, and so on. When looking for the specific determinants of smoking we have investigated variables such as smoking habits of parents and classmates, amount of pocket money, and smoking control measures in schools.

In the mid-1970s the concepts of 'way of life' and 'life style' were ardently debated among Finnish social scientists. The debate evoked our interest in the inter-relationships of health habits and from this one empirical aim of the study was defined '. . . to investigate whether health habits aggregate to renewing and wearing life styles' (The Juvenile Health Habit Study 1979). We took the term life style from the debate of social scientists and operationalized it for our study on the basis of the epidemiological school of thought (Fig. 13.1). Life style was understood as an aggregation of certain types of health habits. Only the habits related to major diseases were regarded as important components of life styles. Life styles were derived from the empirical data by applying various kinds of 'numerical methods'. A typical result of that exercise was a description of three alternative life styles in young people:

- tobacco and alcohol users,
- butter, coffee, and sugar users (mainly children of rural farmers),
- 'healthy' life style (neither tobacco nor alcohol, physically active, good dental hygiene, etc.).

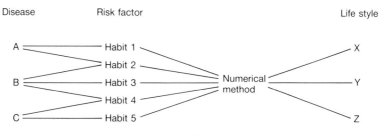

Fig. 13.1.

Trends in health habits

The first results regarding the trends in health habits were available in the autumn of 1977. We compared this data with unpublished data on smoking from a 1973 survey on alcohol use in young people. We found a significant decrease in the prevalence of smoking since 1973 (Rimpela and Eskola 1977). Two years later, in 1979, we demonstrated a further decrease in smoking and the National Board of Health was satisfied with the perfor-mance of its smoking control policy.

In the studies of 1981 to 1985 the results were not as positive for smoking control policy as in 1979 (Fig. 13.2). The prevalence of heavy smokers (10+ cigarettes per day) rose to the level of 1977. In 14-year-old boys it was almost equal to the figures of 1973. The Tobacco Act forbids selling of cigarettes to children who are younger than 16 years. In directives given by the national authorities a strict control of smoking in schools has been emphasized. From 1977 to 1983 there were no obvious changes in purchasing cigarettes nor smoking in schools (Rahkonen and Rimpela 1984). The response rate gradually decreased by nearly 10 per cent from 86–88 per cent in the three

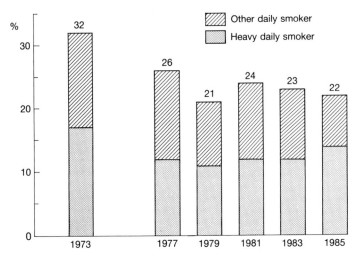

Fig. 13.2.

first surveys to 80 per cent in 1985. Consequently, the real smoking rates in 1985 may be even higher than in 1977.

From the above data we must conclude that the Finnish smoking and health programme was successful in the 1970s, but not in the 1980s. The information about the trends in other health habits opens up new questions. Boys at the age of 14 years seem to be especially prone to unhealthy habits. This subgroup can serve as an example when looking at trends (Fig. 13.3). Since 1977 the use of alcohol has slightly decreased, dental hygiene is improving, and the use of butter and high-fat milk, as well as the use of coffee, have all diminished remarkably. In addition to that data from Fig. 13.3, we can find significant changes in other subgroups. Vitamins and tonics have become popular and the use of p-pills in girls is increasing rapidly (Kosunen *et al*. 1986).

A thorough discussion of the above findings is not necessary here. We want to emphasize the differences between a picture based only on smoking data and the one based upon the trends in several other habits. The resources available, and the administrative and legislative support for the prevention of smoking, have been much greater than for activities related to any other habit listed above. However, from the health point of view the changes in the other health habits have been more positive than the trends in smoking.

Why the smoking policy succeeded in the 1970s but failed in the 1980s is not known. The lesson from our study is that we need a nationwide

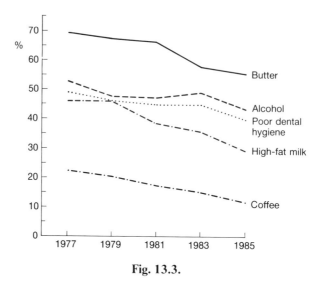

Fig. 13.3.

information system which should cover as many habits and activities of young people as possible. There is also an urgent need for parallel and more specific investigations of what is going on in the world of young people. The smoking control activities cannot be evaluated in isolation, but must be put into the context of young people's social reality. Surveys similar to ours may open new questions, but in the end provide few answers.

New areas of interest

From the point of view of the epidemiological tradition our study was a success. The panel design gave interesting results and we were able to describe formation of smoking habits and point out several determinants of that process (Rimpela 1980). We could demonstrate a strong and obviously causal relationship between smoking and respiratory symptoms as early as the age of 14 to 16 years (Rimpela A. 1982). It has also been possible to evaluate the health hazards of low-tar cigarettes (Rimpela A. and Rimpela M. 1985). Our team has published several reports on the other health habits in local (Rimpela M. *et al*. 1983) and international journals (alcohol: Ahlstrom 1982; dental hygiene: Honkala *et al*. 1984; use of butter and milk: Arttla *et al*. 1986; use of coffee: Hemminki *et al*. 1986).

However, we have not been satisfied with our approach. In each survey we have experimented with new areas of interest. These interests were not derived from a comprehensive conceptual frame but from our attempts to broaden the scope step by step:

Autumn 1977: Dental hygiene.
Spring 1979: Sleeping and perceived tiredness, physical maturation.
Autumn 1979: Psychosomatic symptoms, dating.
Spring 1981: Perceived health, patterns of menstruation, drugs, use of 'junk' food.
Spring 1983: Hopes and fears, perceived threat of war.
Spring 1985: Hobbies, social support, health service use.

Some of the new areas have had an important impact on our conceptual thinking and they will be further discussed.

Health habits v. maturation

In discussion with paediatricians we became interested in the role of physical maturation in the formation of health habits. Literature searches yielded little except a few sporadic comments. We were not able to find any serious study on the role of physical maturation in smoking and use of alcohol. We added a simple question about the age of the first menstrual period into the survey of the spring of 1979. Two years later, in 1981, we found a similar indicator of boys' physical maturation: the age of the first ejaculation.

These questions give an opportunity to classify our respondents into an early, average, and late maturing group. Having a narrow range of the calendar age (ten or fewer consecutive birth days) we demonstrated a strong relationship between physical maturation and several health habits (Table 13.2). This confirms that more emphasis should be put on the process of physical maturation as it is a central phenomenon in the life of boys and girls (Rimpella *et al*. 1986). Measurement of that process should be included in all studies on health behaviour from 10 to 16 years of age.

Table 13.2 Percentage of smokers and alcohol-users among 14-year-old girls by age of menarche

Health habit	Age of menarche				Not occurred
	−11	12	13	14	
Daily smoking	26	14	6	10	6
Alcohol monthly or more often	24	20	15	8	1
(N)	(74)	(68)	(171)	(67)	(67)

Perceived health

When analysing the impact of smoking on respiratory symptoms we wished to enquire into the health status of the respondents. Perceived chronic morbidity and respiratory symptoms were asked from the beginning of the study. In our department we worked in close collaboration with a team investigating the inter-relations between health, occupational strain, and social class. They found that a list of symptoms, derived from the Cornell Medical Index, measured occupational strain (Aro 1981). A literature search showed no population studies on perceived symptoms in adolescents, and we decided to experiment with this instrument in the autumn 1979 survey which was the last survey of our first panel study.

Every fourth boy and more than every third girl reported symptoms (headache, irritability or fits of anger, abdominal pains, nervosity, difficulties in sleeping, etc.) fairly often. More than 10 per cent of the 14-year-olds had one or more symptoms almost every day. The higher prevalence of symptoms in girls was mainly due to menstrual pains. Originally we thought that our instrument measured specific symptoms, whose meaning was dependent on the diseases they were supposed to indicate. But various techniques of the analyses concerning the aggregation of the symptoms did not produce any clear structure. The conclusion was that the sum-index of symptoms indicate a perceived unhealthiness, which in young people is more related to their life situation than to a specific disease.

Those findings gave us a reason to look at our data on morbidity from a new point of view. Besides serving as the dependent variables in studies on respiratory symptoms, they could be understood as independent indicators of perceived health problems. About one in ten 14-year-olds reported one or more chronic diseases or disabilities causing significant limitations to their daily activities. Every third boy and girl reported at least two bouts of influenza during the preceding six months. The common experience of illness episodes was confirmed by the data from the use of medicines. One in three boys and every second girl had used medicines for aches, coughs, fever, or other similar reasons during the preceding month.

The above findings refer to various kinds of specific disorders perceived by the respondents. We have asked a few questions about the perception of their own health in general. The following items were included in the index of general perception of poor health:

- Health in general 'very bad'.
- Physical condition 'very bad'.
- Perceived weight 'very much under/over'.
- Very tired in the daytime.
- Very seldom feel active in the morning.

The main finding was that about 20 per cent of respondents reported one or more of the health problems listed above.

As a summary of our perceived health measurements we conclude that the myth of a 'healthy young generation' is seriously misleading. Perceived symptoms, worries about own health in general and illness episodes are a common experience among school children, who develop very early on their own ways to cope with these problems.

Perceived health vs. health habits

The orientation of studies considering the relation between health and habits usually starts from diseases. Habits are regarded as potential risk factors and the task is to find out the possible causal processes. Such was our framework when trying to find out the role of smoking in young people's respiratory symptoms.

When we demonstrated a strong relationship between the measures of perceived health and harmful health habits (Fig. 13.4), there was no obvious interpretation of that finding. Most of the medically trained health education experts have referred to the harmful consequences of smoking. The opposite interpretation is to understand smoking or use of alcohol as a common coping mechanism among those having poorer health than the average. When dealing with young people the first hypothesis on its own cannot

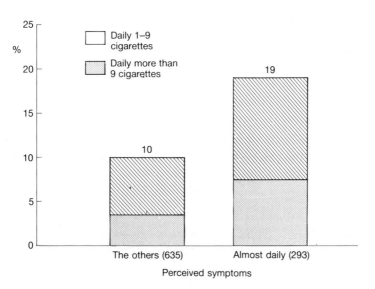

Fig. 13.4.

explain the phenomenon because of the low level of exposure to a harmful agent. The second hypothesis is also too simplistic. Without making any interpretations about the nature of the relationship, the conclusion is that, by the age of 12–14 years, those who perceive a lot of health problems are especially prone to harmful health habits.

The threat of war

The issue of nuclear war was much debated in the Finnish mass media in 1981–1982. One of the hot topics was whether children perceive a serious threat of nuclear war and whether that threat causes any mental disturbances. Once again we faced a situation where plenty of opinions were available but there was no information about the perception of threat and its effects in young people. The survey of 1983 was at this time in preparation and so we added a few questions on hopes and fears in general and about the perceived threat of war (Solantaus *et al*. 1985).

At that time we did not see any immediate association between the original task of our survey and the issue of war. However, when analysing and reporting the results from that area we ran into important conceptual and methodological discussions which can be summarized as follows:

1. What kind of formal and informal criteria do we apply when including some areas of human thinking and action in health behaviour and excluding some other areas from it?
2. What is the role of perceived symptoms and anxiety in health of adolescents: do they indicate good or bad health?
3. Where are the limits of a survey applying mailed questionnaires as a method of data collection?

The term 'health behaviour' is widely used but seldom thoroughly discussed from the conceptual point of view. A typical feature of definitions is that they refer to one's activities in relation to his/her health. When the actions are aiming at strengthening the health of one's family, colleagues, the nation or mankind as a whole, they are labelled as hobbies, party political activities, or humanistic interests. To a health promotion activist a community control programme is still 'a real thing' in comparison with active participation in global health movements. However, the amount of unnecessary diseases and deaths due to famines and wars is certainly higher than those due to coronary heart disease. In the light of this the behaviour related to the global health issues may be regarded as a dimension of health behaviour, along with behaviour related to risk factors of major chronic diseases.

The questions about perceived symptoms were originally supposed to indicate problems in health: the smaller the number of symptoms the healthier the respondent. Later we had to reconsider this interpretation of symptoms. Ability to perceive the changes in the functions of one's own body may be extremely important to the normal development of the body image in adolescence. A similar rethinking also became necessary in the inter-pretation of the meaning of anxiety due to the threat of war. It can be claimed that those who worried about the present world situation are healthier than those who avoid thinking about it (Solantaus and Rimpela 1986). The criteria of health in adolescence cannot be derived only from epidemiological studies on the aetiology of chronic diseases. What is regarded as an unhealthy behaviour from that point of view, may be a healthy reaction in adolescence and important to mental and social maturation. The questions on the threat of war have demonstrated the limits of mailed surveys. Although the percentage of missing answers was low and the results were repeated in independent surveys, qualitative interviews highlighted a classical methodo-logical problem. The survey instrument measured mainly public accounts and described the general climate of opinion, but was not sensitive enough for private accounts. This methodological problem is well known in social sciences (Cornwell 1985) but often ignored in health behaviour research.

Social support

Because of methodological problems we limited the variables describing respondents' social background to those commonly used in epidemiological surveys. In the 1985 survey two questions about the availability of social support were tested. The first one measured the number of good friends and the second one the easiness of talking about things that really bothered the respondent with the parents, siblings, and friends.

The prevalence of perceived symptoms was almost three times higher in those reporting difficulties in discussing things with both parents than in those finding it easy to discuss things with either the mother or father (Fig. 13.5).

When the number of good friends is used as an indicator of social support, the data lead to an unexpected finding: the more social support from friends, the more common is smoking and use of alcohol. This question seems to measure primarily the anticipation of adulthood and independence from the parents' control.

In a bivariate analysis the relationship between health habits and easiness in discussion with parents was not clear. The analysis was then limited to those finding discussion with friends easy and the respondents were classified into three categories according to easiness with parents (easy, mixed, difficult). The percentage of daily smokers was about four times higher in those having difficulties in discussions with their parents than in those having warm relations with their parents (Fig. 13.6).

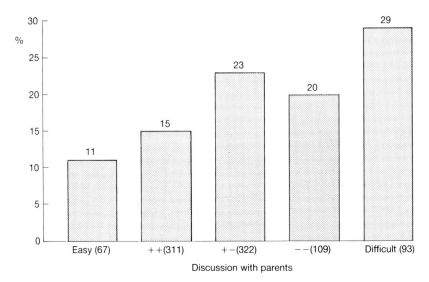

Fig. 13.5.

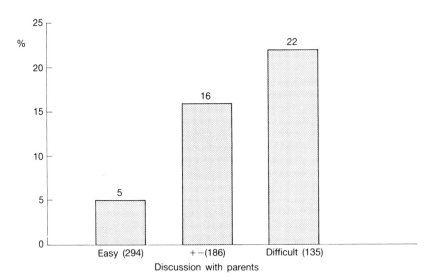

Fig. 13.6.

Although the questions dealing with social support are only rough instruments, they seem to discriminate the smokers from non-smokers better than many of the traditional background variables.

Concluding remarks

The final goal of our study is to develop a nationwide information system to follow up changes in health behaviour of young people. In the beginning there were no serious conceptual problems. The approach of the epidemiological research on diseases was applied to habits. The scope of the study was defined by the administrative interest in smoking and by the aetiological research on chronic diseases which pointed to the habits which were to be regarded as health habits.

Within the past ten years our task has appeared to be much more complex than was expected in the beginning. Our impression is that the development of a health information system has run into a crisis: increasing amounts of data and better technical solutions of data collection and analysis have not solved the most burning problems of health policy. On the contrary, the gap between the world of information systems and the world of everyday health activities is becoming wider and wider.

We have found two issues which are central to attempts to implement a new information system for health promotion:

1. Administrative information systems automatically focus the interests of researchers, planners, decision makers, and mass media people on the issues described in detail in routine documents. Therefore, the best way to ensure a dominant position to some defined issues is to include them in health information systems, while the best way to leave aside the others is to exclude them from the system. The way items are reported as well as the items themselves is crucial.

2. There is an inevitable conflict between the traditional concept of health information systems and the nature of information needed for health promotion. The theory of information systems emphasizes comparability over time and over various social circumstances. A good health information system is static and scientific. The indicators for Health For All are derived from that tradition aiming at a global picture of health developments. In health promotion our target is moving all the time. What is extremely important and measured with a great accuracy today, may be peripheral in ten years' time. The social reality where health promotion should have its effects is changing rapidly. In Finland, a smoker of today is in many ways different from a smoker of the early 1970s. Information needed for health promotion is particular, specific to time, place and social circumstances.

We do not deny the importance of adding new health promotion related items into the existing health information systems. When this is the only development in the field, it may easily postpone the development of those needs of health promotion which are regarded as challenging or repressed interests in our present administration. Besides the small steps within the existing tradition there is an urgent need to develop a new conceptual frame of information systems which fits into the WHO-EURO approach to health promotion.

The evolution of our study reflects the changing realities in Finnish society. In the middle of the 1970s smoking was the health issue. During the past ten years we have added numerous new areas into our study. Afterwards it is easy to see a systematic trend: we were moving from specific disorders towards a more holistic view of health in adolescence and from problems defined by the medical profession to problems perceived as problems by young people themselves. Applying those two dimensions we can demonstrate a typology, which clarifies the limitations of our original approach (Fig. 13.7).

Smoking, use of alcohol, poor dental hygiene, physical inactivity, and the like, are hardly regarded as 'health problems' by young people themselves. They are defined as problems by adults and health professionals. On the other hand, the adolescents report numerous self-defined health problems from chronic diseases to general feeling of poor health and tiredness. They commonly cope with those problems by using medicines. When summarizing the materials collected within ten years we have covered all four types of health problems demonstrated in Fig. 13.6. Due to our limited scope in the beginning of the study, our follow up has been limited to a few habits until now. Our first conclusion that is health information systems on young people should concentrate on self-defined human health problems.

The second conclusion deals with independent variables according to which the changes in health habits are analysed. When the prevalence of smoking is reported by age, sex, place of residence, smoking of parents, smoking of peers, and school performance, the information gives a certain direction to the control activities. When the habits are also related to maturation, perceived health problems, and social support, many new apsects may be taken into account when planning for health promotion. In the beginning of our study a high response rate was emphasized. This was an additional motive to limit the scope of the study. However, the questions which were needed to measure the new areas seemed to fit fairly well into a mailed questionnaire. The factor limiting the study has not been the method as such but our way of defining the scope of the study.

The third conclusion refers to the practical meaning of this exercise. The trends in smoking habits have not been as favourable as we expected when the Tobacco Act was implemented. How is it possible that in a country whose health care system is regarded by WHO as a model for other member countries, where the Tobacco Act is one of the strongest in the world, and

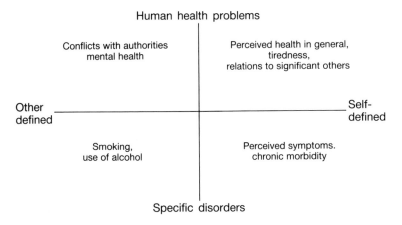

Fig. 13.7.

where one of the most famous health education experiments (The North Karelia Project, see Vartiainen *et al*. 1986) has been carried out, the smoking in young people does not decrease? As our study demonstrates, health promotion activities in Finland are strongly influenced by the school of thought developed within the prevention of chronic diseases. One possible explanation of the slow progress in the prevention of smoking may be this monolithic approach to health education which seems not only to be ineffective but may even be counterproductive among adolescents.

What has been presented above describes an evolution of a particular study programme. Many of our findings and conclusions may not be new to those who have not been influenced by such strong dominant structural interests as we were at the time of starting the study. However, our final conclusion is that the scope of a health information system to follow up changes in health behaviour of young people cannot be derived only from the epidemiological research of major diseases and from administrative interests. If we are not responsive to the needs of young people and problems they regard as important ones, we are selling a product with no use to the consumers. On the other hand, when supporting the physical, mental and social maturation of young people in those areas where they ask for support, the prevention of harmful habits may become easier. The key areas of any information system dealing with the health of young people are:

- process of maturation,
- human relations and social support mechanisms, and
- perceived health, symptoms and disease episodes.

Only a minority of young people are at risk of becoming regular smokers, but everybody has to learn to cope with maturation, human relations, and perceived health problems.

References

Ahlstrom, S. (1982). *Finnish teenagers—how they drink and clash with authority*. Reports from the Social Research Institute of Alcohol Studies, No. 159, Helsinki.

Alford, R. (1975). *Health care politics*. University of Chicago.

Aro, S. (1981). Stress, morbidity and stress-related behaviour. *Scandinavian Journal of Social Medicine* Suppl. 25.

Cornwell, J. (1984). *Hard-earned lives: accounts of health and illness from East London*.

Hemminki, E., Rahkonen, O., Rimpela, A., and Rimpela, M. (1986). Coffee drinking among Finnish youth. Submitted for publication.

Honkala, E., Rimpela, M., and Pasanen, M. (1984). Trends in the development of oral hygiene habits in Finnish adolescents from 1977 to 1981. *Community Dentistry and Oral Epidemiology* **12**, 72–7.

Kosunen, E., Temperi, J., and Rimpela, M. (1986). Ehkaisypillereiden kaytto - 14–18 - vuotiailla tytoilla vuosina 1981–1985. Submitted for publication.

Leppo, K. (1978). Smoking control policy and legislation. *British Medical Journal* **1**, 345–7.

Leppo, K. and Vertio H. (1986). Smoking control in Finland: a case study in policy formulation and implementation. *Health Promotion* **1** (in press).

Prattala, R., Rahkonen, O., and Rimpela, M. (1986). Consumption patterns of critical fat sources among adolescents in 1977–1985. *Nutrition Research* (in press).

Rahkonen, O. and Rimpela, M. (1984). Tobacco in the minds of the adolescents 1977–1983—have the objectives of the Tobacco Act been fulfilled? *The Yearbook of the Health Education Research*. Publications of the National Board of Health. Health education series original reports, No. 5, Helsinki (English summary).

Rimpela, A. (1982). Occurrence of respiratory diseases and symptoms among Finnish youth—a follow up survey. *Acta Paediatrica Scandinavica*. Suppl. 297.

Rimpela, A. and Rimpela, M. (1985). Increased risk of respiratory symptoms in young smokers of low tar cigarettes. *British Medical Journal* **290**, 1461–3.

Rimpela, A. and Teperi, J. (1986). Respiratory symptoms and low-tar smoking—a follow up study. Unpublished manuscript.

Rimpela, M. (1978). Cigarette smoking and public policy. *Scandinavian Journal of Respiratory Diseases* Suppl. 102.

Rimpela, M. (1980). Incidence of smoking among Finnish youth—a follow-up study. *Kansanterveystieteen Julkaisuja*, M 56–80, Tampere (English summary).

Rimpela, M. (1985). From the screening of illnesses to psycho-social support for schoolchildren: a view from Finland. In *New directions in health education* (ed. G. Campbell). Basingstoke, Macmillan.

Rimpela, M. and Eskola, A. (1977). On the study of health habits: smoking habits of the youth as an example. *Sosiologia* **14**, 181–95.

Rimpela, M., Byckling, T., Rahkonen, O., Rimpela, A., and Teperi, J. (1986). Physical maturation as a determinant of young people's health habits. Unpublished manuscript.

Rimpela, M., Rimpela, A., Ahlstrom, S., Honkal, E., Kannas, L., Laasko, L., Paronen, O., Rajala, M., and Telama, R. (1983). *Health habits among Finnish youth. The Juvenile Health Habit Study 1977–1979*. Publications of the National Board of Health, Finland. Health Education Series original reports No. 4, Helsinki (English summary).

Solantaus, T. and Rimpela, M. (1986). Mental health and the threat of nuclear war—a suitable case for treatment? *International Journal of Mental Health* (in press).

Solantaus, T., Rimpela, M., and Rahkonen, O. (1985). Social epidemiology of the experience of threat of war among Finnish youth. *Social Science and Medicine* **21**, 145–51.

Vartiainen, E., Pallonen, U., McAlister, A., Koskela, K., and Puska, P. (1986). Four year follow up results of the smoking prevention program in the North Karelia Youth Project. *Preventive Medicine* **15**, 692–8.

14

Health beliefs and behaviour in the workplace
LAMBERTO BRIZIARELLI

Introduction

The strategy 'health for all by 2000' and the cultural and operative content in the Alma-Ata declaration consider participation of the population—one of its fundamental components—as the central point of health promotion and prevention. However, the two terms are to be kept distinct. Health promotion, far more than prevention, encompasses social actions as a whole and not only health services. Participation becomes an essential condition in workplaces, more than elsewhere, because of their particular characteristics.

For both employees and self-employed workers subjectiveness and personal commitment are essential for: (a) recognizing and analyzing risk factors and conditions; and (b) changing environmental conditions and work organization. This also applies to the changes which have been in progress for some time now in the various work sectors.

As for all environmental problems in workplaces, especially those concerning organization and management, health promotion and participation are not independent variables. They depend on numerous factors which are not completely controllable by health policies, but are determined by the conditions (political, economic, social) of each production or work sector.

Energy policies, the division of labour (national and international), the need for a supply of raw and other production materials, the need for work in general, and the production and technology typologies are all of prime importance in determining the quality and nature of workplaces and organization. However, citizens' and workers' participation is strongly, at times totally, influenced by factors which have little to do with the health objective, such as fear of losing the job, the degree of unionism, the economic position, the state of the market, production ratio, etc.

Although workers' behaviour is essential for health at work, it is well known that they do not always have a positive attitude towards health. Diffuse phenomena like money risk compensation lead to acceptance of working conditions, which have been recognized to be health damaging.

This, without doubt, is to be attributed to the fact that behaviour is the outcome of a myriad of pressure elements which, at work, are stronger and more conditioning than choices available elsewhere.

Given these elements, the objective or value of 'health promotion' tends to fade into the background and is completely forgotten unless, of course, illness, accidents, or even death are caused by the poor conditions.

From this viewpoint, the study of each individual behaviour alone would not enable us to understand the dynamics which occur in a given workplace as a whole. Indeed, behaviour should be considered in relation to the elements which contribute to forming dynamics, whether negative or positive, internal or external.

Behaviour indicators

In order to assess the public health plans, we listed those indicators (Briziarelli and Dirindin 1987) evaluating the positive and negative influences which health intervention exerts on individuals and the community, and the extent to which it determines positive behaviour and attitudes towards health. They include:

1. Specific parameters analysing the effects of education intervention (campaigns, health education for target groups divided according to risk, territory, environment, physiological states, etc.).
2. Parameters singling out how the population may be influenced by health action and the services (behaviour of health pesonnel, ways of providing health care, network of centres, type of health care, characteristics of homogeneity, equality, accessibility, etc.), as well as other actions of the society.

These indicators were divided into three groups: knowledge, attitudes and behaviour.

Knowledge

1. Basic knowledge of health (of one's own body, of the ways and means of protecting health, of health, disease, etc.).
2. Knowledge of risks (general, specific, etc.).
3. Knowledge of services (their functions, the health care to be provided, what is to be expected, etc.) and regulations.
4. Knowledge of the dangerous effects of some medical care.

Attitudes

1. Towards oneself (use of the body; life styles—food, tobacco, drug and alcohol use, leisure time; in certain conditions—lactation, pregnancy, old age, etc.).
2. Towards the services—satisfaction or dissatisfaction: acceptability, accessibility, suitability.

3. Towards the components: health care (quality, quantity), health personnel, individual services, individual centres.
4. Towards health procedures.

Behaviour

1. Indicative of risk exposure in everyday life, work, leisure time (use of protective means and regulations, etc.).
2. Predictive of health promotion (personal hygiene, self-mediation, use of body, time for physical activity and rest, participation in prevention activity, defending the environment, etc.).
3. Estimative of the service activities and the efficacy of health care (use, non-use or mal-use; use of alternative services; resorting to private health care; following through medical orders; carrying out duty and social or work roles, etc.).

For the analysis and description of behaviour in work environments we will refer to this framework. The elements related to knowledge, attitudes and behaviour are described and considered, both potentially and currently, as different phases of a single process pertaining to participation.

Worker's attitudes, knowledge and behaviour

From our own experience and the data in the literature a series of indications arise which are neither uniform nor consistent. We shall attempt to outline the common elements and the discrepancies.

Apart from the influence of promotional factors and the demand brought about by the presence of health services, lay people generally have a preventive attitude towards health. This also applies to workers, and is expressed very clearly when speaking of safeguarding health in factories (Baroncini 1985; Invernizzi 1981). It is referred to as the 'workers' model' (on which our personal experience is based), and it has been largely experimented and applied in other countries besides Italy. Its validity is now recognized in scientific circles.

This model moves beyond the 'safeguarding of occupational diseases and the accidents at work', typical of traditional occupational medicine.

Nevertheless, their attitude does not always correspond to their behaviour. Often workers behave positively in workplaces; outside, however, they behave similarly to others as regards both self-inflicted risk factors and the health services.

Their submissiveness towards health personnel and their impassive acceptance of the lack of consideration in health institutions are tantamount to intransigent attitudes and behaviour towards their adversary during labour disputes (strikes, picketing).

This contradiction can be attributed to the differences found in individual and collective behaviour and attitudes, as was clearly depicted in research we carried out in a large factory in central Italy (Mori 1979). In fact, the social control exerted by the group over the individual when expressing forms of behaviour, even in the presence of the diverse knowledge and attitudes of the individuals, is well known.

Numerous differences are found amongst workers and vary according to their production sector, work relationships and their position in the hierarchy.

Workers employed in industry show a more positive attitude and behaviour towards health than the self-employed (artisans, farmers). This is not necessarily due to the risk factors, since in some areas under study the working conditions were worse in the latter group (Biocca and Schirripa 1981).

Amongst factory workers there are great differences between sectors—first come those in the chemical and metallurgical and mechanical industries and, last, the building industry.

Clerks' and executives' knowledge and attitudes are often better than the factory workers'. This is most likely due to the level of education, as shown in a recent survey carried out in our region (Umbria) (Briziarelli *et al*. 1985). It is also known that the behaviour of these subjects in safeguarding health in workplaces is far less positive than that of the factory workers, contrary to what occurs in other environments. The survey revealed that they had a much higher level of knowledge and behaviour on ecological themes than on work matters.

Exact knowledge on risk factors at work was relatively low, although it was higher in blue-collar workers and managers than in artisans and low white-collar workers. It was better in people with higher school qualifications and young people.

The sexes also differed considerably, in that many more males show positive attitudes and behaviour in workplaces than females (Baroncini 1985; Briziarelli *et al.* 1983).

However, when considering service and office workers the attitude and behaviour of women is similar to that of men. This is particularly true for cadres and executives (Invernizzi 1981), while female office workers holding lower appointments behave less positively.

Similar observations, even though relating to another sector, have been made by numerous authors, who have shown the great influence of social isolation, low socio-economic levels, education (Phillips and Brennan 1976), occupation, position held (Huttner 1976), and participation in social life (Huttner 1976; Jonkers 1981) on women's knowledge, attitudes, and behaviour.

One author (Zincone 1983) refers to a 'social and political' weakness of women caused by a 'two-phase handicap':

1. Family work reduces the possibility of women working outside due (*a*) to their stronger affective link to the house, and (*b*) to the weight of family work.
2. Women's work in the family frees men of the household activities and thus reinforces the male manpower in the labour market.

Others (Black 1972) found women lack ambition and 'career orientation'. Another (Sullerot 1978) referred to women as being less ambitious at work than men for 'biological reasons'.

Age was found to play an important role in determining the knowledge and behaviour of workers towards health. It also seems to cancel out the differences between white- and blue-collar workers. Invernizzi (1981) found a considerable difference in the unionization of older workers (63 per cent— blue-collar, 26 per cent—white-collar workers) and also in thinking about fighting forms for bargaining, whereas the younger workers showed the same amount of unionization and no differences in struggle forms.

Within the same group of workers behavioural differences are found in the various phases of labour history, as can be seen by the varying forms of monetary compensation and with the fall in demand for better environmental and work conditions.

Some authors (Candela and Guidetti 1985) refer to a great initiative of health education amongst working women without bargaining issues due to the serious economic crisis of 1981–82.

In the behaviour of factory workers and workers in general, a number of differences can be seen between collective action for general purposes and individual action, or that of small groups, in a given workplace.

Italy is a typical example—the factory workers' movement during the late 1960s and early 1970s brought about profound changes in the country's legislative, contractual, and organizatory order in the health system and other sectors of society.

Law no. 300 (Statute of Workers' Rights), law no. 833 which institutes the NHS, the regional laws which control a diffuse network of services for safeguarding health in workplaces on a preventive basis, the collective labour agreements with their strong preventive implications are all the direct consequence of the workers' behaviour.

Even before 1970, most industry agreements included:

1. The workers' right to have an expert of their choice control risk factors.
2. The right to have adequate check-ups.
3. The Unions' right to be informed of the production cycles, technologies and the substances used in the manufacturing processes.
4. The right to be consulted for all development and diversification plans.
5. The right to hold a personal health and risk card.

6. The right to have access to other informative means, such as the records of environmental data and biostatistic data.
7. The right to call on the public health services, or other services of the workers' choice, for environmental control and medical check-ups in workplaces.

In each single company, and in entire production sections, even better results were obtained with negotiations. Profound changes and improvements were brought about in work conditions.

The great nationwide upheaval (only local in some sections) involving all sectors of the society, did not reflect the diffuse prevention culture, and was not put into general practice. Nor were the advantages fully used which the State laws and contract regulations put at the workers' disposal.

The agricultural, handicrafts, and building sectors and a number of textile industries (mainly female labour) only partially adopted, if at all, what had become a routine procedure in many other workplaces.

Generally speaking, most workers then had, and still have, the attitude (and behaviour) to delegate their concerns to trades unions and public health services.

To sum up, we are faced with a very well-defined picture of situations which vary so much that we cannot refer to an overall behaviour of workers.

Our experience has shown that there are two distinct groups of subjects: (*a*) workers employed in industry, including managers and clerks, whose knowledge, attitudes, and behaviour towards health are quite positive; and (*b*) services and public administration workers, including self-employed agriculture and handicraft workers, and female labour, whose knowledge, attitudes, and behaviour are less positive.

As a whole, the workers' knowledge of risk factors present at work is quite good, unlike their knowledge and use of protective means. Their knowledge of the services and regulations which should guarantee the safeguarding of health in workplaces, is also rather poor; however, it is generally better than that of other citizens. Younger people's knowledge is better than older people's, males more than females.

The workers' attitude as a whole is preventive and positive towards the health services and health personnel. Their attitude towards union organizations varies greatly according to sector, age, sex, and the region of residence.

Behaviour is often different from knowledge and attitudes, and at times is difficult to evaluate.

In extremely unfavourable environmental and work conditions, absenteeism becomes the only alternative for workers when other means of prevention are lacking. Their positive attitude towards doctors may be triggered by the possibility of attaining easy medical certification, which would guarantee their absenteeism.

Not being able to change the situation the monetary compensation for risks becomes a means of taking advantage in a dangerous environment.

Factors influencing behaviour

From what has been revealed to date, it seems evident that:

1. As observed in various sectors of society, precise correlations do not exist between knowledge and attitudes on the one hand, and behaviour on the other; furthermore, this discordance is present also within homogeneous work sectors.
2. There are considerable differences between behaviour in the workplaces and outside.
3. Individual behaviour differs greatly from collective behaviour, especially in small social groups.
4. Workers' behaviour regarding the promotion and safeguarding of health in workplaces, is influenced by a series of diverse factors which are not necessarily correlated with the health need.
5. The type of work done, the relevant sector, and the position held assume great importance in determining behaviour and undoubtedly influence behaviour related not only to the work environment (such as smoking, drinking, eating habits, etc.).

   Factors positively or negatively influencing the workers' behaviour may be broadly divided into two groups: (*a*) factors intrinsic to workers and their condition, which could also be called individual or subjective; and (*b*) extrinsic factors, deriving from conditions outside the specific health or working context, which may also be described as environmental or of social origin.

   The intrinsic factors include:

- age: younger people generally behave more positively towards health;
- sex: women behave much less positively than men;
- civil state: married couples show a less positive behaviour;
- work sector: which weighs heavily on behaviour towards health;
- residence: generally in southern regions behaviour is far less positive than in the north;
- social condition/class: the lumpenproletariat accept work in any conditions.

   The extrinsic factors include:

- overall economic situation: changes are usually more difficult during recessions;
- degree of development: in underdeveloped areas changes are always difficult;

- structure of the firm: decentralization of production and the multi-national structure make negotiations complex;
- general political situation: in non-democratic states, with secret Mafia-like forms of power, negotiations are generally repressed, if not completely impeded.

Undoubtedly the latter group of factors is much more important than the former in influencing, if not completely determining, behaviour. Likewise, the factors in the second group are often the cause of the differences ascribed to the first group.

The differences attributable to sex (i.e. the generally less positive attitude of women workers) are closely linked to the cultural and social conditioning (Rudas 1982) which has determined the role of women—the division of household jobs and other work, bringing up children, different education according to sex, the political role of women, etc.

A behavioural analysis model

On the grounds of the classification presented earlier, the following list of indicators is proposed to analyse workers' behaviour.

Knowledge
1. General, i.e. related not only to the work environment.
2. Specific.

- Of risk factors present in the work environment.
- Of the materials used.
- Of working processes, including work organization.
- Of protective means.
- Of safety rules.
- Of regulations, workers' rights, contract institutions.

Attitudes
1. General, i.e. related not only to the work environment.
2. Specific.

- Towards the unions and the company's representative body.
- Towards the ways and means of changing the environment or work organization.
- Towards the chiefs.
- Towards work.

Behaviour

1. General, i.e. related not only to the work environment.
2. Specific.

- Participation, together with experts, in activities to protect the environment.
- Participation in activities proposed by the unions, such as assemblies, manifestations, strikes, picketing.
- Union membership.
- Behaviour at work, e.g. doing overtime, accepting shifts, etc.

However, apart from the analysis of indicators and their subjective precursors (knowledge and attitudes), research will have to be directed towards singling out external factors from which behaviour stems.

The analysis of external or environmental factors (social, economic, political, structural, group, etc.) is indeed the sole element which may provide information on the actual reasons for certain behaviour, and thus indicate the type of intervention for health promotion, prevention, and health education.

These three integrative terms are mentioned separately in order to refer to the three different groups who intervene in the overall process of health promotion: citizens, experts and health workers in general, and the decision makers.

It is equally evident that the indications defining their particular roles should be found in research, through singling out the different times and levels of intervention.

This chapter is not meant to deal with the methodological aspects in detail, so we shall limit ourselves to a few brief indications. The models used are extremely varied and diverse, and depend upon the situations encountered.

In our surveys we have used means and tools of various kinds, from questionnaire-guided interviews with individuals and groups, personal interviews and discussions in homogeneous groups, to questionnaires filled out by the individual worker and by groups, or by the delegate or shop steward.

These tools may be used separately, according to the situation, but, at times, more than one may be used for the same survey (for instance, individual interviews and group discussions).

From our own experience we have noted that more detailed, and at times more precise, information is usually obtained in group discussions rather than in interviews or individual questionnaires.

Finally,with regard to health promotion, from a conceptual viewpoint and considering the suitable form of intervention, I feel some specific points may be put forward.

The promotion of health in workplaces cannot be exclusively assigned to the health services and/or occupational medicine. A wider spread of intervention is required and should involve other sectors of public intervention, such as social services and structures, social security institutes, and formative structures.

These are, indeed, of primary importance in harmonizing the conditions of the workers with those of the citizens, and in cancelling the overall negative effects which hinder the fulfilment of one of man's fundamental needs—work.

The health promotion of workers depends only to a certain extent on health policies and activity; it mainly lies in the general policies which determine work relations, the means and quality of production, work conditions, and environment.

This evidently calls for a drastic quality change in the policies of the States and public authorities—to place health at the centre of the development process—an objective which combines the actions of decision makers, the services, individuals, and the community.

References

Baroncini, P. (1985). Crisi operaia tra Taylorismo e automazione (Crisis of blue-collar workers between Taylorism and automation). *ISPE, Quaderni* **34**, 35.

Biocca, M. and Schirripa, P. (1981). Esperienze di lotta contro la nocività in alcune aziende italiane tra il 1965 e il 1980 (Fight against nocivity in some Italian firms between 1965 and 1980). *CENSAPI, Roma*.

Black, G. S. (1972). A theory of political ambition: career advice and the role of structural incentives. *American Political Science Review* **116**, 000.

Briziarelli, L. and Dirindin, N. (1988). An indicator system for the evaluation of public health programs: the case of the Region of Piedmont. In *Indicators and trends in health and health care* (ed. D. Schwefel). Springer-Verlag, Berlin.

Briziarelli, L., Minelli, L., Modolo, M. A., Mori, M., Panella, V., and Ranocchia, D. (1985). People's health and health attitudes and knowledge in Umbria. Paper presented at the 12th World Conference on Health Education, Dublin.

Briziarelli, L., Modolo, M. A., Mori, M., and Panella, V. (1983). Primo approccio ad una classificazione degli indicatori di comportamento (An approach to the classification of behavioural indicators). In Atti del 31° Congresso Nazionale di Igiene, Ancona.

Candela, S. and Guidetti, P. (1985). I rischi da lavoro in gravidanza (Work risks during pregnancy). *Regione Emilia Romagna, Contributi*, No. 11, 000.

Huttner, I. (1976). Social aspect of the participation of women in preventive screening for cancer of uterine cervix in the GDR. *UICC Technical Report Series* **24**, 32.

Invernizzi, E. (1981). Impiegati e operai: verso una nuova 'Classe di Lavoratori' (White and blue collar workers: towards a new 'Working Class'). *Quaderni di Rassegna Sindacale* **89**, 25.

Jonkers, R. (1981). Knowledge, attitudes and behavioural intentions as indicators of coping with breast cancer. In *Health education and media* (eds. D. S. Leathar, G. B. Hastings and J. K. Davies), p. 411. Pergamon Press, Oxford.

Mori, M., Briziarelli, L. and Marcuccini, A. M. (1979). Condizione operaia e salute (workers' state and health). *Regione Umbria, Quaderni, Serie Sanità*, No. 1, Perugia.

Phillips, A. J. and Brennan, M. E. (1976). The reaction of Canadian women to the Pap test and breast self-examination. *UICC Technical Report Series* **18**, 24.

Rudas, N. (1982). Aspetti psicologici dell'esperienza lavorativa (psychological aspects of working experience). In *La parità tra lavoratori e lavoratrici e la tutela della salute*. Ist. Ital. di Medicina Sociale, Roma.

Sullerot, E. (1978). *Il fenomeno donna*. Sansoni, Fl.

Torti, M. T. (1979). *Lavoro e nocività* (*Work and nocivity*). Ghiron, Genova.

Zincone, G. (1983). L'accesso delle donne alle arene decisionali: una ricerca europa (women's access to the decision making area: a European survey). *Quaderni di Rassegna Sindacale* **105**, 84.

15

Health promotion and the concept of community

JOHN ASHTON

Introduction

Health promotion is acquiring a considerable momentum as part of the emerging new public health movement. Central to the concept is a focus on populations defined in terms of their community affinity. However, there are many concepts of community and the field is paved with ambiguity and misconception. The World Health Organization framework has helped to provide valuable cohesion. It is now becoming clear that parallel research methodologies need to be developed which, like health promotion itself, are diverse but complementary. Health promotion is ultimately about holism and synthesis and this will need to be reflected in these methodologies.

The problem of definition

According to the British Faculty of Community Medicine, community medicine is that branch of medical practice which is concerned to promote the health of human communities. It is assumed that what is meant by 'community' is understood. Yet, according to Phillips and Le Gates (1981) there are at least 90 definitions of 'community' in sociology.

As a native of Liverpool it is appropriate for me to be thought of to a certain extent as a member of the community of Liverpool, a citizen of that city. Yet Liverpool itself is actually a city of villages and estates with very different identities; some of these are readily defined as such while others only emerge to a non-villager on growing awareness of the subtle boundaries which exist between one part of an apparently homogeneous district and another. Where do I stand if I live in one place and work in another?

The Faculty of Community Medicine definition has its origins in the administrative medicine of the public services and seems to imply that 'the community' is a kind of geographical black box fixed in time and space and containing all kinds of assumed structures and functions such as 'the family' and 'opinion formers and decision takers'. A somewhat more operational definition, although also based on geography, was that adopted by the

Peckham Pioneer Health Centre in determining who was eligible for membership—those within pram-walking distance, the equivalent of one mile (Ashton 1977). This geographical concept of community is reflected in one of the three main dictionary definitions:

'A body of people living in one place or district or country and considered as a whole' (*The Oxford Dictionary*, 1983).

Yet I, as a citizen of Liverpool and a resident of one of its villages, am also a member of a range of other communities in addition to a rather large if dispersed 'community' of family and kin—the medical community, the university community, social ecologists, and the international communities of health promoters and family planners. Each of these communities of affinity is responsible in some way for influences on my assumptions and values, experiences and lifestyle, and in the midst of this is my core identity as an individual; all matters of central interest in any consideration of the 'health field' in which pro- and anti-health forces interact. According to Hancock and Duhl (1986) the meaning of community in all the varying senses hinges on the notions of 'togetherness and sharing'. The other two main dictionary definitions 'a group with common interests or origins' and 'fellowship, being alike in some way, community of interest' thereby become subsumed into a concept which may only sometimes be bound in time and space but which may frequently be more approximately considered as some kind of network (discussion document, WHO Copenhagen, 1984). Habitat, work, play, class, race, kin, hobbies, religion, and personality are just a few of the 'communities of interest' which must therefore attract the attention of the health promotion researcher.

The task of health promotion and emerging patterns of activity— experience in one region

Health promotion is the process of enabling people to increase control over, and to improve, their health (Ashton 1986). It is an ambitious concept which is centrally an ecological one and one which recognizes that health is much more than the result of health services and health care. Health is seen as 'a resource for everyday life, not the objective of living' (discussion document, WHO Copenhagen, 1984).

As described by the European Region of the World Health Organization there are five key principles to health promotion:

1. Health promotion involves the population as a whole in the context of their everyday life, rather than focusing on people at risk for specific diseases.
2. Health promotion is directed towards action on the determinants or causes of health.

3. Health promotion combines diverse but complementary methods or approaches.
4. Health promotion aims particularly at effective and concrete public participation.
5. Health professionals—particularly in primary health care—have an important role in nurturing and enabling health promotion.

According to Kickbusch, health promotion is essentially about creating a new public health. This will involve changing public and corporate policies to make them conducive to health and involves re-orientating health services to the maintenance and development of health in the population (Kickbusch 1985). Health promotion strategies stress the constant interaction between ways of life and healthy public policy, and therefore health policy must cover not only planning for the provision of services but planning for health (Ashton 1986). The key recurring themes in the emerging literature on health promotion are the emphasis on participation and multi-sectoral approaches.

Three years' experience of developing a health promotion strategy in one British region has helped to clarify a number of the issues which are central to this process of developing a new public health (Ashton and Seymour 1985; Ashton *et al*. 1986).

The strategy which has been developed in the Mersey region has three main strands:

1. Agenda setting.
2. Consciousness raising.
3. Development of models of good practice.

Agenda setting

Since 1974, British health authorities have had the responsibility for what was called preventive medicine prior to the development of the health promotion concept. In recognizing the importance of including health promotion in the planning process of the health bureaucracy, a first step was to ensure that the scope and nature of health promotion was understood by decision takers within the bureaucracies. This was addressed by the production of a community diagnosis which was launched at a regionwide conference, the production of a chapter on health promotion in the regional strategic plan and the inclusion of the subject in the review process, whereby each health district is monitored on its policies and progress (Ashton 1984, 1985). Each district was expected to develop its own plan for health promotion based on the activities of a multi-disciplinary health promotion team (Ashton 1982). This process, which is clearly a top–down one, has been most effective in ensuring that health districts accord appropriate weight to the development of health promotion. However, it has opened up an immense field for research in terms of what has actually happened and why and what effect district policies are having.

Consciousness raising

The deliberate adoption of a high profile for health promotion at a regional level, with the active creation of Health News and a pro-active approach to the media, has been coupled with a large-scale job creation scheme—the health buses; with the aid of the five buses and 130 previously unemployed young people on the buses, 300 000 people have had personal contact with the health promotion unit in a two-year period, and 50 000 have had a personal fitness test carried out complete with life style assessment and recommendations. The twin aims of the bus project have been job creation/personal development for the young unemployed and mass consciousness raising among the general public on health issues—the bottom-up approach.

Models of good practice

In order to overcome the negativism which commonly seems to accompany attempts at innovation in Britain, locally based models of good practice have been developed. One of the most useful of these appears to be the health centre-based Health and Recreation Team (HART) which has as its brief to facilitate the networking of health and recreation facilities at the local level and to bring about a re-orientation of services where appropriate. The project has apparently successfully tapped the enormous interest in physical recreation and been able to connect this interest up with physical and human resources—the integrated approach.

The experience of developing these strands has helped to identify the following needs:

The need for positive indicators in place of negative ones and for qualitative and small area data   The Mersey Strategy has 12 priority topics derived from epidemiological analysis and review of current health-promotion literature:

(*a*)   planned parenthood,
(*b*)   control of sexually transmitted disease,
(*c*)   antenatal care including genetic screening,
(*d*)   improved child health and increased immunization uptake,
(*e*)   the prevention of death and disability from accidents and environmental causes,
(*f*)   improved dental health,
(*g*)   some specific aspects of life style related to premature death (including diet, exercise, stress, tobacco, alcohol, and drugs),

(*h*)   the effective control of high blood pressure,

(*i*)   early detection of cancer,

(*j*)   reduction in disability in the elderly,

(*k*)   dignity and comfort at the time of death,

(*l*)   a healthy mind and healthy body—positive health especially as it relates to a health strategy for young people.

Most of the currently available data in relation to these topics is medical/ pathological or administrative in nature, whereas health promotion needs to focus on the healthy rather than the sick and on processes rather than organization. Such data that is available is difficult to relate to 'community' denominators; there is a particular deficiency of special survey data at small area level and 'soft' descriptive data at any level.

Indicators of participation and intersectoral function do not currently exist and those of networking, empowerment, and community morale are illustrative of others which need to be developed. One of the lessons to be learned from the history of public health is the motivating power of information if it relates to people at their own local level and there is a pressing need to produce this information for health promotion.

The need to focus on contexts as well as people   An important concern of critical observers of the new public health in recent years has been the danger of victim blaming (Labonte and Penfold 1981; Hancock 1986). This is well illustrated by a recent survey of nutritional knowledge and shopping behaviour in five wards of Liverpool. In the study, 100 people were interviewed from each of the five wards as they left their local supermarket where they had been shopping. Four of the wards were in the inner city or outer city estates with high levels of public housing and were characterized by high unemployment, a low proportion of owner occupiers, and a number of other indicators of social and material disadvantage. The fifth ward was chosen for comparison because it was in an affluent part of the city with no apparent indication of deprivation. Participants were questioned as to their knowledge of nutrition related to heart disease and as to the shopping which they had purchased for their families. Despite the fairly crude nature of the survey a consistent picture emerged with those people who lived in the favoured part of the city being much further along the path towards the implementation of coronary prevention recommendations for themselves and their families, than those from the other four wards. The advantaged shopper profile could be described as salt conscious, high fibre, low fat consuming, non-smoking, as compared with the disadvantaged shoppers' salt-adding, low fibre, high fat, and smoking. What became clear in the course of this survey was the restriction on the exercise of healthy choices and behaviour which comes not only from ignorance but also from having low income, living in a part of the city served by low-cost, low-quality super-markets with poor food-labelling and having no private transport with which to take advantage of shopping facilities elsewhere. Clearly the mesh of factors—knowledge and attitudes, income, geography, transport, and retail choice—is the real focus for research in this area. Such a focus would need to be able to accommodate idiosyncratic cultural or subcultural practices, e.g. salt or sugar added to porridge among Scots or the continued familiarity with the uses of pulses to make soup as with older people.

Doing things from where people are—people-centred health promotion   The traditional model of public health is a paternalistic one. Having identified hazards to the public health, the Medical Officer of Health had access to the whole panoply of public health legislation with which to enforce his recommended action. In turn this has led to a tendency with the new public health to attempt to travel the same route. Prescription based on epidemiological analysis tends to be the logical outcome of medically-based health promotion programmes. Such programmes tend to be top–down rather than bottom– up and vertical rather than horizontal. Vertical programmes, such as specific coronary prevention initiatives, impose a disease-based model on everyday life and life styles. The alternative is support for processes which integrate different aspects of a healthy life-style at the community level, but which start from everybody's own interest in the health of themselves, their family, and their social group, the organizational counterpart being primary health care.

In this emerging dichotomy of approaches important research needs to be done to clarify the processes at work. The questions include: whose priority? whose initiative? why and how? and, particularly, whether real participation and intersectoral collaboration was to be found. Horizontal, ecological approaches to epidemiological, behavioural, and sociological–anthropological research need to be developed.

An emerging style is that of social entrepreneurism and opportunism—for health promoters to be on the look-out for opportunities to work with communities who are at a stage of development where they are willing to pick up some concepts and work with them. This seems to be very different from the medicocentric imperialism which has hitherto dominated; its overwhelming characteristic is partnership, acting with or for, rather than on.

Recent examples within the Mersey Region include collaboration with a womens' health action group who were compaigning for a health centre, and with a community organization wishing to create work by putting people and derelict land together in an inner city area of high unemployment. In the first instance statistical analysis to support the case seemed to be an appropriate response; in the second, assistance to obtain funding for a feasibility study of a community business based on urban horticulture.

The need for true stories John Snow and the Broad Street Pump, Karelia and Stanford, the Welsh Heart Project, and the Liverpool project on teenage pregnancy, the folk stories of public health, and the parables for training new generations of workers; yet what was the truth in each case? Who did what, when? and why? really? Did the initiative really come from the 'community' or were professionals involved in a softening-up process first. Did they give history a shove? Why was this project funded now but not a similar project sooner or later, or a project on a different topic but with similar methodology? So we really do need true stories—yet, if we had really known the truth would the inspiration provided by some of the myths have led to real achievements?

Health-promoting capabilities of a community It seems likely that the prerequisite for effective community participation in health promotion includes the availability of accurate information and the possibility of remedial action at the right time and in the right place. How were these conditions created? We need to find ways in which to describe communities which take account of community empowerment and self-esteem, the collective and social equivalents of concepts which we understand well for the individual. Erikson's developmental approach to the tasks of maturation seems pertinent here, as does the whole field of work on locus of control (Erikson 1967; Slater 1976; Beal 1985). Do we have adequate typologies for describing the stage of development for communities in their involvement with the processes of health promotion or do we need to create new ones?

What makes a healty city/school/family/institution? Does the triage model have any value here in appraisal? And what is it about some communities which makes them adventurous and risk-taking, willing to innovate and experiment, whilst others are conservative, defensive, even paranoid?

An understanding of these and related phenomena is essential if we are to make sense of health promotion initiatives and of their evaluation. A structural model of the human eco-system suitable to accommodate dimensions of process has been put forward by Hancock and Perkins of the Department of Public Health in the City of Toronto (Fig. 15.1).

Perspectives

Placing the new public health in some kind of historical context is a priority. It is clear that an understanding of history can, of itself, be beneficial not solely because the political dimensions and options become clearer in the collective arena but because, on a personal level, an understanding of social history is one with which people readily identify and which can be motivating and energizing. A recent example of this is the use of a four-generation account of a Baltic island family as recorded by a district nurse and midwife; this has

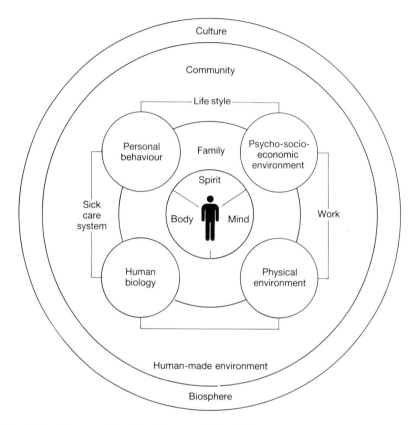

Fig. 15.1 The mandala of health—a model of the human eco-system (Hancock and Perkins—by kind permission of the Department of Public Health, City of Toronto.

been extensively used to open up discussion in the Swedish programme designed to increase understanding of sexuality and personal relations, and reduce the incidence of teenage pregnancy. A further example would be the presentation derived from the National Advisory Committee on Nutrition Education (NACNE) report for use at the Liverpool International Garden Festival in 1984 (Health Education Council, 1984). This material recounted the changes in family eating habits during the past 200 years and their relationship to the increasing incidence of heart disease; the presentation drew on documentary evidence derived from household budgets.

Just as the historical perspectives can throw light on health promotion issues at a community and family level, so can projection of demographic change linked to behavioural and social science knowledge give some understanding of what we can expect in the future. How do the children of the

Welfare State differ from teen cohorts before and since? (Ashton 1983). What mega values and mega behaviours can be predicted from a knowledge of birth order, family size, cohort affinity, and experience? Does Garreau's version of neo-regionalism based on affinity groups and networks have any general application? (Garreau 1981). Is the medium now indeed the message; are there communities whose affinities are wholly or mostly defined by telecommunication and travel linkages; has the global village really arrived? (McCluhan 1964).

To link in, describe and, if possible, quantify some of these concepts, social psychology, anthropology, and ethnology, will presumably be of important service together with the new ecological epidemiology.

Dilemmas and pitfalls

For the public health activist restraint can be a difficult discipline. Yet it is probable that the most effective health promoting initiatives will come from within communities rather than from outside them. The dilemma of the researcher in becoming too closely identified with intervenors remains real in health promotion as in any service-related research activity. The desire to achieve some prior stated outcome is particularly strong in vertical programmes funded by external sources. Those responsible for health promotion face the challenging task of synthesizing the horizontal with the vertical in keeping with the communities' own priorities. Measures of process may be a much more acceptable evaluation than the attempt to define some hard end-point which is epidemiologically respectable.

A question which arises for those involved in comparisons between communities is whether there has to be ontogeny. Do communities at different stages of development have to repeat each others' mistakes? What are the factors which facilitate short-cutting and transference of community learning? There is a danger too of fantasies of perfect communities—pre-Raphaelite innocence, the village before Adam; such comparative ideal types cannot be left unchallenged. The inner city is not the only place with problems; how does one measure and balance up anonymity/freedom with total knownness/claustrophobic oversight? How does one measure optimal mess and uncertainty?

Appropriate methodologies and techniques: the need for synthesis

By definition health promotion combines diverse but complementary methods and approaches; it therefore requires research methodologies which are also diverse but complementary (WHO Copenhagen 1984). The polarization of quantitative and qualitative methods advocates is unhelpful here as elsewhere; what is needed is synthesis. Techniques may be available from elsewhere, particularly from behavioural science as developed in relation to psychotherapies, or from market research as a means of developing cybernetic community communication. There is a need for community-centred as opposed to researcher- or individual-centred measures, and proxy measures are likely to be important because of the difficulty in obtaining direct measures which are valid in their own right, e.g. is the suicide rate an appropriate indirect measure of community stress suitable to research the stress component of coronary heart disease in a population?

Participation/engagement by individuals and groups is clearly an area which could benefit from the research methods developed in relation to clinical (especially child) psychiatry, and similar social–psychological measures need to be derived to explore those dimensions of health-promoting interaction which are related to power and gender.

One specific area for development would appear to be that of geometric modelling. The problem of ontogenesis has already been referred to; it should be possible to produce graphic typologies of communities experiencing particular health-related changes, e.g. urbanization and increasing standard of living leading to increased heart disease death rates followed by societal change resulting in reduced risk factor levels. If there are natural histories to such societal changes then different time, period, and cohort patterns may be interpreted in a meaningful way in the light of specific health promotion initiatives. The paradigm-changed sexual behaviour/increased unintended pregnancy rates/changed contraceptive behaviour/reduced unintended pregnancy rates provides a similar, familiar pattern, the time course of which seems to vary between countries and depends upon the social attitudes towards teenagers and sex, and the willingness of adults to respond to the needs of young people (Jones *et al.* 1985). It may be gratifying for public health personnel to make their reputations by riding the downward wave of epidemics but it may not be the most appropriate use of public resources.

Above all health promotion is about synthesis; about holism rather than reductionism; and about reconciling the various artificial dichotomies which have been constructed as partial explanations of our realities. In the same way that those active in supporting the processes of health promotion need to network their efforts and move freely between geographical, historical, and personal senses of community, research workers in this field need to shadow those networks and find parallel methods.

In their recent review of the literature on cities for the WHO Healthy Cities project, Hancock and Duhl (1986) suggest 11 parameters as worthy of consideration in the appraisal of a city:

1. A clean, safe, high quality physical environment (including housing quality).

2. An eco-system which is stable now and sustainable in the long term.
3. A strong, mutually-supportive and non-exploitative community.
4. A high degree of public participation in and control over the decisions affecting one's life, health, and well-being.
5. The meeting of basic needs (food, water, shelter, income, safety, work) for all the city's people.
6. Access to a wide variety of experience and resources with the possibility of multiple contacts, interaction, and communication.
7. A diverse vital and innovative city economy.
8. Encouragement of connectedness with the past, with the cultural and biological heritage, and with other groups and individuals.
9. A city form that is compatible with and enhances the above parameters and behaviours.
10. An optimum of appropriate public health and sick care services accessible to all.
11. High health status (both high positive health status and low disease status).

The healthy city concept is a powerful one because it provides a unifying framework in which to consider health promotion—the challenge to research now is to produce a parallel response.

References

Ashton, J. R. (1977). The Peckham pioneer health centre: a reappraisal. *Community Health* **8**, 132–7.
Ashton, J. R. (1982). Towards prevention—an outline plan for the development of health promotion teams. *Community Medicine* **4**, 231.
Ashton, J. (1983). Children of the Welfare State. *New Society* **64**, 109–10.
Ashton, J. (1984). *Health in Mersey—a review*. University of Liverpool, Department of Community Health.
Ashton, J. R. (1985). Health in Mersey—an exercise in community diagnosis. *Health Education Journal* **44**, 178–80.
Ashton, J. (1986). *Promoting health in three nations*. Kings Fund, London.
Ashton, J. and Seymour, H. (1985). An approach to health promotion in one region. *Community Medicine* **7**, 78–86.
Ashton, J., Seymour, H., Ingledew, D., Ireland, R., Hopley, E., Parry, A., Ryan, J. and Holbourn, A. (1986). Promoting the New Public Health in Mersey. *Health Education Journal* **45**, 174–9.
Beal, N. (ed.) (1985). *Repertory grid techniques and personal construction*. Croom Helm, London.
Brackpool, J., Ramharry, S., and Ashton, J. (1985). *Shopping and coronary prevention in Liverpool*. Liverpool University, Department of Community Health.
Erikson, E. H. (1967). *Childhood and society*. Pelican, London.
Garreau, J. (1981). *The nine nations of North America*. Avon Publishers, Canada.

Hancock, T. (1986). Lalonde and beyond: looking back at 'a new perspective on health of Canadians'. Personal communication.

Hancock, T. and Duhl, L. J. (1986). Healthy cities: promoting health in the urban context. A background paper for the Healthy Cities Symposium, Portugal, 7–11 April 1986. WHO, Copenhagen.

Health Education Council (1984). Proposals for nutritional guidelines for health education in Britain (NACNE) report.

Jones E. F. *et al.* (1985). Teenage pregnancy in developed countries: determinants and policy implications. *Family Planning Perspectives* **17**, 53–63.

Kickbusch, I. (1985). Health promotion—the move towards a new public health. Personal communication.

Labonte, R. and Penfold, S. (1981). Canadian perspectives in health promotion: a critique. *Health Education*, April 4–9.

Larsson, B. (1978). A Gotland family. Socialstyrelsen namnd for halsoupplysning, S-1-6 30, Stockholm, Sweden.

McCluhan, M. (1964). *The Global Village*. Quoted in *McLuhan* by J. Miller. Fontana, Modern Masters (1971).

Phillips, E. B. and Le Gates, R. T. (1981). *City lights; an introduction to urban studies*. Oxford University Press, New York.

Slater, P. (ed.) (1976). *The measurement of intrapersonal space by grid techniques*. John Wiley & Sons Ltd., Chichester.

The Oxford Dictionary (1983). Oxford University Press.

WHO Copenhagen (1984). Health Promotion, a discussion document on the concepts and principles (ICP/HSR 602).

SECTION E

The application of research in health behaviour

INTRODUCTION

Robert Anderson

There is not only an intellectual market for knowledge on health and human behaviour; growing numbers of people are employed to manage and apply such research or elements of it. The practical interests in health behaviour research reflect the growing importance for health policy of the promotion of life styles conducive to health. So, information is required for monitoring trends in health behaviour, for identifying health problems and social groups in particular need, for the design and planning and evaluation of social and health interventions, for developing new ideas, and for giving the community a voice in health matters.

It may be that, compared with the university departments, the needs for information in the applied market are different and more prosaic. The practical demands of developing and implementing programmes influence the nature of the research undertaken. From the currently available research the question addressed here is what we can learn about and for the plethora of life style surveys. Studies are presented here from three countries, two at national (Canada, Scotland) and one at regional (Madrid) level. The national experiences are relatively long-standing and their development reflects the uses for which the research is designed. The regional initiative is a recent development and the authors document some of the many financial, organizational, and structural problems in establishing systematic health behaviour research.

Martinez and Peruga discuss the contribution of health behaviour research in regional health planning and how this can be organized for maximum effect. They reflect upon the context of research in a country which is in transition from an authoritarian to a democratic state, with an associated decentralization of planning and need for information at regional level. However, the regional initiative, like its national counterpart, is oriented to strategic planning and the monitoring of longer-term objectives—this demands measurable outcomes based upon data collected routinely in the information system. In practice, as the authors note, about two-thirds of the national research in public health is concentrated in activities in the Madrid region. Data collection focuses upon specific health behaviours such as smoking, and alcohol and drug consumption. An institute has been created to enhance the application of research in regional health planning. The institute is structured to integrate several functions by combining diverse roles: in research, the development of health promotion strategies, co-ordination of action for health promotion, and not least the development of appropriate personnel for both general health services and health promotion.

For Canada, Rootman describes how research has been applied in the development and evaluation of many health promotion programmes. There are numerous health behaviour surveys,many repeated at regular intervals. However, as the author notes, it is always very difficult as a researcher to know to what extent the research has been usefully applied because there is generally little feedback. Rootman shows how the results of research have been used to re-orientate the health system to respond to new problems. He also shows how results can be disseminated widely to inform the public, stimulating interest, enabling action, and generating momentum for health promotion. To engage the widest possible audience researchers have used news-sheets, articles, the press, and consultations in the community. These multiple methods are illustrated as mechanisms or levers for stimulating action. There are examples from Canada of relatively novel data-collection strategies including, for example, the training of volunteers in workplace programmes who conduct the research and use the results to mobilize their local communities into action. The author documents how, possibly especially in a very large country like Canada, local research is important and how the monitoring of behaviour in relation to local health promotion programmes might contribute to evaluation. However, like other authors, he notes deficiencies in the use of health behaviour resarch including the under-application of available research, shortage of comparable area data and gaps in the links between research and planning.

John Davies illustrates the Scottish experience with many examples from a wide range of settings, often funded through the Scottish Health Education Group. He indicates that health behaviour research is beginning to move from exclusive focus on risks for specific diseases towards factors influencing good health and personal development. Social psychological studies of risk behaviour contributed many ideas applicable to the methods and content of communications. However, the use made by health educators was *ad hoc* and unsystematic. This deficiency was due in part to a lack of infrastructure for regular routine surveys, especially those which provided useful data at the level of Scotland within the United Kingdom; there was also a lack of involvement of practitioners in the study design and there were few long-established researchers in the field. These problems reflected a certain tension between the demands of science (academia) and those of practice, even though many studies were funded specifically to support the development, application, and evaluation of programmes. There have been many difficulties, especially in the identification of and implementation of appropriate methodologies for evaluation; considerable potential still exists for linking academic units to work closely with health promotion and health education agencies.

All three papers point to the need to establish organizational and structural links between researchers and programme or policy people. There is still inadequate longer term co-ordination of research and planning. In practical terms the effectiveness of research and the application of its results would, it appears, be facilitated by greater attention to protocols that can be applied at local level permitting comparison of health behaviours between different areas.

16

The autonomous region of Madrid

ROSE MARTINEZ and ARMANDO PERUGA

The aim of this chapter is to present some general considerations regarding the role of health-behaviour research in regional health planning activities. In order to present the subject matter within a contextual framework, reference will be made to the health-planning activities now being developed in the autonomous region of Madrid in Spain. Beforehand, however, it is considered important to provide a brief exposition on the present socio-political context which characterizes Spain as a society in change, the present status of health-behaviour research, and regional health planning in the autonomous region of Madrid.

Context

A brief description of the Spanish socio-political context must make reference to the situation of change which has been occurring during the past ten years and which is fundamentally characterized by the transition from an authoritarian state to that of a democratic state. This transition has had a notable influence upon social behaviour as well as the general organization of Spanish society. With respect to the latter, it should be emphasized that this intense decentralization process has led to the constitution of 17 autonomous regions with their respective parliaments and governments.

Although the process of decentralization cannot be considered as completed, its influence is already far-reaching. For example, the changes in the health sector are quite noticeable, allowing for the first time reference to the existence of regional health authorities with responsibilities for the promotion of health and the prevention of disease among its inhabitants. A long road must be covered, however, before the transformation of the health system is completed and resembles the new health system proposed by the General Health Law which was recently approved by the national parliament. The General Health Law allows for fundamental changes to be made in the health system which are in line with the spirit of Health for All by the Year 2000.

Among the changes occurring and expected in the future, changes in the mode of financing the health system are not expected to be made. Presently, the health system is funded in a large part by the social security system (national financing) and in a smaller part by the autonomous government (regional financing). This fragmentation in the financing system is directly related to the existence of various health service networks within the region with different sources of financing. Thus, it appears that a diversified network providing health care assistance will continue to exist; a network, on the one hand, under the auspices of the national social security system and, on the other, under the auspices of the autonomous governments. This circumstance is mentioned because it has and will continue to exercise an influence upon the health-planning activities in the region.

Characteristics of regional health planning in Madrid

At the present moment, the type of health planning which is being carried out in the region is characterized as strategic and global and not solely operative and partial. Its strategic nature is defined as short- and long-term planning within a defined health policy framework which is, in consequence, directly related to the political element of decision making. In practice, however, strategic planning is often used as a technical instrument responding to the political situation rather than at the request of the administrative–operative organization (organs of administration) for the formulation of objectives and strategies which permit the development of health and social welfare policy which the regional Health Ministry has outlined.

With respect to the global nature of health planning, it is understood that planning activities should take into consideration both health and social services, thus providing a sense of wholeness to social policy. In general, this global nature of health planning contemplates as an objective of its action the individual in an integral manner, as well as the co-ordination of health resources and services.

It can also be understood by global planning that activities should be directed at the entire public health system and should not be limited to particular sub-networks of resources and services. This means that within the health sector, the planning activities which are carried out should refer not only to the regional health network but should also include the national social security network. This characteristic of the global nature of health planning is an expression of the political will to unify the existing networks as stipulated in the socialist programme and to provide an integrated and coherent system of services.

Based upon this strategic and global perspective of health planning, the regional health planning organization has four functions:

1. To establish health and social welfare objectives which are defined and measurable, within a specified time period, indicating the priority of each

one with respect to criteria based upon the needs of the population, and determined by the necessary research activities.

2. To collect, analyse, distribute, and generate, in each case, the information necessary for executing the aforementioned function, and thus for producing a routine information system from the planning organization to the administrative organs, and vice versa.
3. To establish the manner by which the planning objectives will be reached through the formulation of strategies and specific goals for each one of the objectives; and to serve as the administrative organs to operationalize the programming of these goals through the deployment of human, material, and economic resources in order to realize the proposed activities.
4. To evaluate programmes and services, from the point of view of their impact and cost-benefit. And with reference to the administrative organs, to participate in the evaluation of the productivity, output, and cost-effectiveness.

These functions are now in the initial phase of development and are experiencing a difficult time in taking root in a political culture which does not have a long tradition in health planning.

A view of health research activities

During the year 1985, Spain dedicated 0.5 per cent of its gross national product to all research and development activities (Maravall 1985). This implies a cost of $8 per inhabitant per year. This expenditure compares to an average expenditure of 1.5 per cent of the gross national product of the OECD countries.

The number of researchers registered in the last census carried out by the Department of Research Policy of the National Ministry of Education and Science is calculated to be 20.2 per 100 000 inhabitants. This compares to 120 researchers per 100 000 inhabitants in the European Economic Community. With respect to the health field, 1500 researchers were registered in the 1980 census as carrying out health-related research, although other non-census sources estimate the true figure to be close to approximately 3000 (the discrepancy in figures may reflect a high level of non-responses especially in the private sector). Of those identified as health researchers, about half are working within the region of Madrid; however, only 32 of these are reported to be carrying out public health-related research.

With respect to the financing of health research, two main sources exist: the Commission on Research and Technology (CAICYT), which funds various types of research, and the Fund for Health Research (FISSS) which funds only health-related research projects. Both of these sources contributed to the seven million dollars which were spent on the financing of health research projects in 1981. Thirty four per cent of these funds were designated to universities, 11 per cent to hospitals of the social security system and the rest to other institutions.

In 1981, in the region of Madrid, a total of 276 research projects were funded out of the 392 projects presented nationally to the two funding sources. This implies that approximately 70 per cent of the projects and 69 per cent of the funds were designated to the region of Madrid (Marquez-Montez and Monteaguado 1985).

In general, the situation of health research in Spain is less developed than in other European countries. However, it should be acknowledged that most of the health-research activities are concentrated in the region of Madrid. With respect to the situation of research in public health-related topics (excluding biomedical, clinical, and laboratory research) the situation is estimated to be far worse although the actual volume of research activities in this area has not been quantified.

In 1984 an attempt was made to modify the research priorities in health by changing the balance of funds available for research in public health-related topics versus that available for biomedical and clinical research. The outcome of this attempt resulted in failure. Only 400 projects were presented during the funding request period with a value of 16 000 000 dollars; however, only 200 000 dollars of the requested funds were granted.

With respect to the carrying out of health-behaviour research, it is difficult to estimate at this time the total number of investigators working in this area in the region of Madrid. However, several research projects which gather information on health behaviours are being carried out by the Regional Institute for Studies of Health and Social Welfare, a branch of the Regional Health Ministry. Some of these current research projects include: a study on the prevalence of alcohol consumption in the region—this study gathers data on alcohol consumption, drug consumption, smoking behaviour, and life style; a study on the needs of the elderly which will also provide some data on life style variables; and a study on health services utilization which will provide information on preventive health care services utilization. In other regions health-behaviour research projects are being conducted, such as in the Basque Country and Barcelona City where regional or local health surveys are done which include items to identify specific health behaviours, especially those related to the consumption of alcohol, drugs, and tobacco.

Role of health-behaviour research in regional health planning

Having presented an overview of the health-behaviour research and health-planning activities in the region of Madrid, it can be seen that these activities are still in an initial phase of development. For this reason it is appropriate to reflect upon the role that health-behaviour research can play in regional health planning in order to develop working propositions for the near future. Furthermore, it is necessary to reflect upon the links which serve to integrate health-behaviour research and planning for their mutual benefit.

It is important to recognize that health-behaviour research plays a fundamental role in the design phase of regional health planning, the development phase, as well as in its implementation phase intended to promote the health of the community and to prevent ill-health. The links between the two activities of health planning and health-behaviour research may be several, among which the following can be considered.

1. The application of knowledge regarding health behaviour.
2. The development of human resources for the implementation of health-promotion programmes and research in health behaviour.
3. The co-ordination of institutions or sectors, not solely health-related ones.

The idea of the administration of health behaviour knowledge refers to its transit between the knowledge produced and the knowledge applied to planning. This idea of the administration of health behaviour knowledge leads not only to a reflection upon the applicability of scientific knowledge regarding health behaviours (and in consequence the research priorities), but also to a reflection upon the organization of the regional health administration.

In this respect the region of Madrid through its Regional Health Ministry has created an institute, the Regional Institute for Studies on Health and Social Welfare, which is organized to enhance the transmission of knowledge produced on health behaviours into an application in health planning. The Regional Institute combines the functions of regional health planning, the development of research activities and the co-ordination of peripheral research activities, and the development of human resources. The fact that a single organization has the responsibility for producing the knowledge on health behaviours, responsibility for setting the priorities and strategies for health promotion, and the development of human resources for carrying out these strategies is undoubtedly a positive factor, particularly if this body also has responsibilities over other sectors such as social services, as occurs in this case.

These functions were designated through the legal framework created for the division of responsibilities between regional and central governments. Nevertheless, this organizational scheme is being used by health planners for enhancing the administration of health behaviour knowledge primarily in the design phase of regional health planning.

In Fig. 16.1, taken from Lopez-Acuña and Romero (1984), the complex relationships between the health-behaviour knowledge produced and applied in health-promotion programmes can be considered. As can be seen,

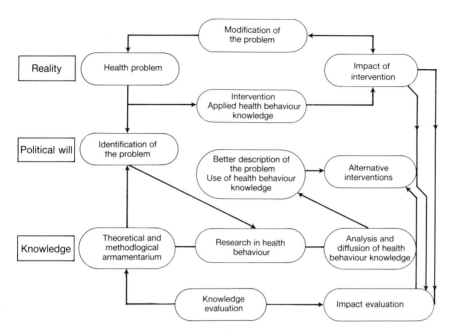

Fig. 16.1 Relationship between the production of health-behaviour knowledge and the procedures for intervention—modified from Lopez-Acuña and Romero (1984).

the identification of the problems and their prioritization, an essential task of planning in the design phase, requires the condition of an adequate amount of political support and the connection between knowledge and reality. It is at this level where planning receives as much from investigation which will permit it to convert this investigation into action. This influence of health-behaviour research upon health planning may be exercised in the definition of general health objectives for all of the region as well as in the formulation of specific objectives for health promotion. In no other way can the necessary interface between planning and investigation be constructed. However, before arriving at this point of interface, it is necessary that the knowledge produced be analysed before establishing priorities and strategies, in order to determine the best characterization of the existing health problems.

At this point the formulation of priorities and alternative strategies of intervention need the contribution of six areas of knowledge in health behaviour, which according to McAlister *et al.* (1982), include the following:

1. The role that preventive services play in the detection of individuals with an abnormal risk.

2. Information necessary for health education.
3. Techniques of persuasion to motivate people to take healthy action.
4. Techniques for acquisition of self-control skills.
5. Availability of community organization to provide social support.
6. Potential for the creation of opportunities for changed health behaviours through environmental changes.

The need to administer knowledge as well as the production of knowledge and the administration of programmes requires the existence of adequate human resources at the regional level. This circumstance demands the collaboration and co-ordination between different administrative institutions and academic institutions. In this sense, the Regional Institute of Studies is in the process of developing a conjoint programme for training with one of the main universities in Madrid. This is considered an innovative experience given that it is the first time that the integration of teaching and research and services is made. In addition, such a programme also allows for the definition of new profiles for health professionals which are based upon actual needs. This last point emphasizes the great importance and need for the training of not only general personnel but also those specialized in the area of health behaviour research and health promotion.

In summary and conclusion, the considerations presented up to this point are indicative of the existing need to link health behaviour research and planning for health promotion and of the possible means of aiding this interface. These considerations have also served to shed some light upon the dilemmas faced by the health administration of Madrid as the authority responsible for the promotion of health in the region.

References

Lopez-Acuña, D. and Romero, A. (1984). Perspectiva de la investigación epidemiológica en el control y vigilancia de los enfermedades. *Salud Pública de Mexico* **26**, 281–96.

McAlister, A. *et al* (1982). Theory and action for health promotion: illustration from the North Karelia Project. *American Journal of Public Health* **72**, 51–3.

Maravall, J. M. (1985). La reforma del sistema ciencia-tecnología ante la crisis. *Mundo Científico* (*La Recherche*) **46**, 445–451.

Marquez-Montes, J. and Monteaguado, J. L. (1985). Tecnología y salud bases para una planifación en ingeniería clinica, investigación y desarrollo industrial. *Informes Tecnicos*, Instituto Regional de Estudios Consejería de Salud y Bienestar Social, Madrid.

17

The Canadian experience

IRVING ROOTMAN

Introduction

In the past 15 years there have been numerous Canadian studies of health behaviours. Some of the better known ones are the Nutrition Canada Survey, the Canada Health Survey, the Canada Fitness Survey, and the Canada Health Knowledge Survey. But how useful have these studies been in developing and monitoring programmes to promote health?

Unfortunately, answering this qustion definitively is impossible for any one individual without actually carrying out a study themselves. This is because information about the use of studies usually remains hidden within the organizations which carry out and use them.

However, it is possible for an individual to report on how such studies have been used by their own organization or by others with which they have close contact. Thus, the author of this chapter can, with some confidence, report on the use of study findings by the Canadian federal government's Health Promotion Directorate. Fortunately, this Directorate is the main body at the national level in Canada concerned with and responsible for health promotion programming. Thus, the use of findings of studies by the Directorate is likely to give a reasonable idea of how such findings are used and are likely to be used in the future in health promotion programming in Canada.

The health promotion directorate

The Health Promotion Directorate was established in 1978 as a response to the much acclaimed report entitled *A New Perspective on the Health of Canadians* which had been issued four years earlier by the Honourable Marc Lalonde (1974) who was at that time Canada's Minister of Health and Welfare. One of the reasons why the Lalonde report was so well received in Canada itself was because the dissemination of the results of studies of health behaviours had helped to prepare the groundwork for its acceptance. The Nutrition Canada Survey, for instance, which had been released six months before the report, had shown that half of Canadian adults were overweight because of low levels of physical activity. Similarly, just four months before the report, the LeDain Commission of Inquiry into the Non-medical Use of Drugs had, on the basis of their studies, identified alcohol use as Canada's most serious drug problem. Be that as it may, it took four years to establish a unit at the national level to give some visible expression to the health promotion philosophy put forward in the Lalonde report.

This unit was composed of elements of six groups located in various parts of the Department of Health and Welfare, the largest one being the Non-medical use of Drugs Directorate. Since its establishment, the Directorate has passed through a number of phases. The results of research have been used in each of these phases but are now beginning to assume more importance than they have in the past, as we are currently in a re-analysis phase in preparation for a serious attempt by the new Canadian government to move forward in the field of health promotion, which will be based on the European office of WHO's definition of health promotion as 'the process of enabling people to increase control over and improve their health' and the principles that flow from this definition (European Office of WHO 1984).

Uses of research

Given this context, how has the Health Promotion Directorate used the results of research on health behaviours in health promotion programming?

It will be noted that research has been used for more than developing and monitoring programmes, although these two uses have certainly been of prime importance.

Informing people

The findings of research have, for instance, been used extensively in informing the public and health workers about health issues. The Directorate regularly disseminates the results of studies on health behaviour. For instance, a series of one-page 'fact sheets' have been produced to present the key results of studies such as the Canada Health Survey (Health and Welfare Canada and Statistics Canada 1981), in a form that will be usable by people working in the field of health promotion. These fact sheets have been distributed with our publication *Health Promotion* (formerly *Health Education*) which is sent to over 10 000 health professionals in Canada. A recent readership survey of the magazine found that the fact sheets were considered to be among the more useful parts of the publication (COGEM Inc. 1984). The fact sheets are also distributed in response to frequent inquiries for statistical information which we receive from the press and the public.

Health promotion itself is also used as a vehicle for disseminating information about the results of Canadian studies on health behaviours. A research column summarizing recent Canadian health promotion studies is published in each issue and there are often special stories on significant studies thought to be of interest to health promotion workers. Again, the research column was considered to be very useful by the readers of the publication in the readership survey (COGEM Inc. 1984).

In addition, the Directorate publishes reports on specific studies or syntheses of the results of various studies. An example of the former is a recently published report of the smoking habits of young people in the Northwest Territories which found that the rates of smoking were among the highest in the world for the age group studied (Millar and Van Rensburg 1983). This report, in addition to providing interesting information to the public, has been used as a basis for stimulating action in the Northwest Territories to deal with smoking among young people as well as for modifying existing resources to fit the unique circumstances of that region.

An example of a report drawing information from various sources is *Alcohol in Canada* which synthesized information on alcohol consumption, problems, and treatment from surveys, other studies, and existing reporting systems (Working Group on Alcohol Statistics 1984). In addition to summarizing the information contained in these sources, the report also contained original analyses particularly of data in the Canadian Health Survey. The report was released at a meeting of the Canada Addictions Foundation, a national non-governmental organization which deals with alcohol problems in Canada, and received widespread national coverage in the electronic and print media. It has subsequently been distributed through our own Directorate and the provincial government bodies responsible for alcohol and drug programmes. Thus, it has reached people working in the alcohol and drug field and also the general public. A recently completed evaluation of resource materials produced by our department for use by provincial addictions agencies, found *Alcohol in Canada* to be one of the most widely used and the resource was given highest priority for updating.

Finally, the results of research are disseminated to the public by press releases, ministerial press conferences, and other means. Thus, it is quite clear that one important use made of health behaviour research in Canada is that of informing people. Such a use is entirely consistent with the European definition of health promotion in that information *per se* is undeniably an important means of *enabling* people to take appropriate action regarding their health and the health of their fellow citizens.

Stimulating action

A second use which is also consistent with this definition is to *stimulate appropriate action*. Such action can be stimulated at a variety of levels.

An example of a recent attempt to stimulate action at the provincial level in Canada using research as a lever is the Canada Health Knowledge Survey (King *et al.* 1984). This survey, carried out in 1982, involved giving a self-administered questionnaire to a provincially representative sample of about 30 000 Canadian school children. The results were not only widely reported in the press but consultations were also held in all provinces and territories between the authors of the study, Directorate staff, and key people in the school health field. To date, the consultations appear to have contributed to changes in school health policies, development of school health programmes, establishment of university courses on school health, and the formation of advocacy groups for school health in a number of jurisdictions. We intend to carry out a follow-up study to find out if there are any improvements in students' health knowledge as a result of these actions.

An example of the use of research to stimulate action at the local level is a project called Mental Health in the Workplace which is being carried out by the Canadian Mental Health Association (1984) with the support of the Directorate's Contribution fund. As part of the first phase of this project, volunteers in five pilot communities carried out a telephone and a key informant survey to assess the needs of their communities in relation to mental health and the opportunities for promoting mental health through the workplace. These surveys have been instrumental in mobilizing the communities to take advantage of the opportunities for promoting mental health through the workplace, although it is too soon to say what kind of an impact their activities might have, the example shows volunteers can in fact be trained to do research and that the results of research can stimulate action at the community level. We thus expect to use such approaches more often in the field of health promotion in Canada.

Having made the point that health behaviour research can be used for important purposes other than programme development and monitoring, we can turn to discussing these two uses, as they are the main foci of this chapter.

Developing programmes

There is no question that research on health behaviours has been used to develop the Health Promotion Directorate's programmes. In fact, it is increasingly difficult to find a Directorate programme, resource, or brochure that does not make extensive use of existing research. One study for example that was extremely important in the development of our 'generation of non-smokers programme' was a national survey of young people and parents carried out in 1981 (Goldfarb Consultants 1981a).

The survey, which was conducted by a major Canadian consulting firm, was designed to assess the public's receptiveness to the generation of non-smokers concept and to determine how the programme could best be delivered. It involved face-to-face interviews with a national sample of about 1000 parents of children under the age of 18 and 400 young people aged 10–18.

The following were among the major findings.

1. Overall, people had a positive reaction to the concept 'toward a generation of non-smoking Canadians'. The vast majority of both parents (89 per cent) and young people (90 per cent) felt it was a good idea. In particular, non-smokers and quitters felt the concept was positive.
2. The general attitude among parents (53 per cent) and even more so among young people (64 per cent) was that Health and Welfare Canada should be doing more to promote non-smoking.
3. People perceived the concept to be education-oriented more than legislation-oriented. That is, they felt the concept implied promoting the benefits of not smoking rather than trying to pass legislation regulating advertising and sale of cigarettes.
4. People expected that the government should promote the concept through television programmes and commercials, general advertising, and in the schools.
5. The overall feeling was that a wide variety of people and organizations should be involved in the communication of this concept.
6. Nearly half of smoking parents and smoking young people said they started smoking because they wanted to be accepted, to be part of the crowd. That is, smoking parents and young people perceived smoking to be socially acceptable behaviour.
7. Young females (42 per cent) were more likely than males (30 per cent) to say they were smoking more, while males were more likely to be smoking less (30 per cent versus 20 per cent) than six months earlier. That is, frequency of smoking appeared to be increasing among young females.
8. The majority of smoking parents (63 per cent) said they did not feel their smoking was a behavioural role model for children. That is, most parents who smoke tend to feel their behaviour does *not* influence their children's behaviours.
9. There was a tendency among non-smokers to feel they were part of a minority of Canadians as opposed to a majority. That is, there was a significant number of non-smokers (50 per cent) who felt the majority of Canadians were smokers.

While this summary of findings does not do justice to the richness of the study and its results, it is suggestive of implications which might be, and in fact have been, important in the development of the generation programme. For instance, the first two findings convinced the people in charge of planning the programme that the public was supportive both of the idea and the role of the federal government in promoting it, and therefore that the programme should proceed. Similarly, the third, fourth, and fifth findings suggested acceptable ways for the federal government to proceed: through television programmes and commercials, general advertising, and in the schools; through educational rather than legislative strategies; and through involving a wide variety of people and organizations. And indeed the subsequent programme used all of these means. Finally, the rest of the findings suggested what some of the content and foci of the programme might be: the need to present a strong image of young non-smokers; the need to give special emphasis to females in the advertisements and other parts of the programme; the need to convince parents of their importance as role models; and the need to try to change the perception of non-smokers that they were a minority. The programme has pursued all of these latter directions with the possible exception of an emphasis on parents as role models, a direction which it is likely to pursue in the future. Thus, this study has been useful in a variety of ways in developing the 'generation of non-smokers programme' and it is anticipted that it will continue to be useful in this regard.

Another study which also was useful in the development of this programme was a qualitative study (Goldfarb Consultants 1981b). In this case, 16 focus groups were conducted in four cities in order to test the campaign approach with teenagers and their parents. Among other things, the focus groups convinced the programme planners that the overall approach would work and that the campaign should proceed. On the other hand, it suggested that more emphasis should be put on the fact line, that the music should be clearer and that commercials on subjects other than the ones tested should be developed. All of these suggestions were implemented.

There are many other examples that could be given of the use of research studies in the development of health promotion programmes within the Health Promotion Directorate and other bodies responsible for health promotion programmes in Canada. However, the ones that have been cited perhaps will suffice in convincing the reader that such research can indeed be used in many ways in the development of health promotion programmes: it can be used to convince programmers and funders of the need for programmes; it can suggest approaches for carrying them out; it can suggest possible content and foci; and it can suggest ways of improving their quality and effectiveness.

Monitoring programmes

As is the case with research to develop programmes, there are many examples of how health behaviour has been used to monitor health promotion programmes in Canada. One with perhaps the longest history is the Smoking Habits of Canadians Survey. This survey was initiated in 1984 by the newly established federal government Smoking and Health Program. It was done by Statistics Canada, the national statistical agency, as a supplementary part of one of its monthly Labour Force Surveys, which is the largest continuous household survey in Canada. It involved obtaining data through interviewing a representative sample of almost 60 000 Canadians.

The first findings of this survey received considerable attention from planners and the public, as previous estimates of smoking activity in Canada had been based on cigarette and tobacco sales rather than on population surveys (Health and Welfare Canada 1983). This 1984 survey established non-smoking as the norm in Canada. However, the results represented an anomaly created by the widespread temporary reduction in smoking after the release of the Surgeon General's report in the United States. It was therefore not used as a basis for monitoring future smoking trends. Rather, the survey which was carried out in the following year was used as a baseline. Since that time, the survey has been repeated approximately every two years, the most recent one taking place in December 1983 (Jossa 1985).

Over this time period, the survey has been used to monitor levels of smoking in the Canadian population as a whole and in particular sub-groups of the population. Its results have been eagerly awaited by people working in the smoking field as well as by voluntary organizations, the press, and the general public. Results have been widely used as one important indicator of the relative success of efforts to reduce smoking in Canada, although other indicators, such as tobacco sales, have been used as well. The findings have also been used to identify particular target groups requiring special attention. For instance, the consistent findings that smoking rates are higher in Quebec than in the rest of the country has led to disproportionate investment of media and other programme resources in that province. Similarly, the findings that the decline in regular smoking among males was relatively greater than that among females (18 per cent versus 3 per cent) over the period 1965–1981, that there was an increase in smoking prevalence rates among women aged 20–24 in two provinces, and that the increase in proportion of regular heavy smokers (smoking over 25 cigarettes per day) between 1970 and 1981 was greater among females than among males (64 per cent versus 24 per cent) helped to convince programmers to pay more attention to females in their programming.

The smoking survey has also been used to help evaluate a specific programme intervention. The programme called 'Time to Quit' involved the distribution of a self-help booklet, a series of television programmes and a community guide for local programme organizers. A pilot study to test the full programme was carried out in Winnipeg in November 1982. Because of the large size of the Labour Force Survey sample it was possible to derive reliable estimates of the prevalence of smoking in Winnipeg as well as a control city, Edmonton, both before and after the campaign. That is, the Labour Force Survey on smoking was used as part of a quasi-experimental design (Millar and Bartlett 1985) to evaluate the impact of the 'Time to Quit' programme.

It was found that between 1981 and 1983 there was a 16.5 per cent decrease in smoking in the test community. The expected annual decline of regular smokers in Winnipeg based on the trend between 1977 and 1981 was about 1 per cent per annum whereas the actual decline was about 3 per cent per annum. This was twice the decline observed in Edmonton. These findings helped the programme organizers conclude that the programme had indeed been successful in reducing smoking in the target population. Thus, the survey which had been designed to monitor smoking patterns of Canadians as a whole, because of the large sample size, was able to be used for evaluation purposes without additional cost.

It should be mentioned, however, that other approaches were used as well in the evaluation of the programme. These included an experimental study of the efficacy of the booklet itself, a panel study of regular smokers in the pilot and control communities, and a participant observation study of community processes. Taken together, these studies provided a comprehensive set of findings which led to specific recommendations for the improvement of the programme. The overall evaluation is described in detail in a recently released report (Millar and Bartlett 1985).

In addition to the Labour Force Survey on Smoking, the Health Promotion Directorate has carried out other studies to monitor its programmes. A current example is a survey to monitor the impact of our three media campaigns Garceau 1985). This survey, conducted each February since 1983, involves interviewing and giving a self-administered questionnaire to a nationally representative sample of young Canadians who form the target groups for the campaigns. Questions are designed to measure their awareness of the campaigns, their knowledge about the issues covered in the campaigns, their attitudes regarding these issues, and their health behaviours. The survey is used not only to measure the achievement of the campaign goals but also to provide an understanding of changes in the social environment in which these campaigns are taking place. As a result of being aware of the findings of this survey, changes have been made in the content and direction of these campaigns by programme officers.

Although the examples of the Labour Force Survey and our media tracking survey may not be typical of studies to monitor health promotion programmes in Canada or elsewhere, they do provide concrete illustration of the usefulness of such studies.

Deficiencies in use of health promotion research in Canada

On the basis of the last section, one might conclude that research has been used extensively in Canada at the national health level for developing and monitoring health promotion programmes as well as for other purposes. While this is so, there remains considerable scope for improvement, inasmuch as there are some deficiencies in the conduct and use of health behaviour research for programme development. Among the key ones are the under-utilization of existing research, the shortage of comparable subnational data, and an absence of comprehensive long-term planning.

Under-utilization of existing research

An example of the under-utilization of existing research is use of the Canada Health Survey (CHS). This survey was carried out jointly by Health and Welfare Canada and Statistics Canada in 1978/79. At considerable expense, health status and health behaviour data were obtained from a nationally representative sample of about 17 000 Canadians. An official report was published in 1981 (Health and Welfare Canada and Statistics Canada 1981) and several papers, some of which have been published (Collishaw and Myers 1984; McDowell and Praught 1982) were subsequently produced. The information has also been disseminated to the public health professional community in Canada and elsewhere. However, information from the CHS has not been used to any significant degree in the development and monitoring of the Health Promotion Directorate programmes. Nor has it been used extensively in the development and monitoring of other health promotion programmes in Canada.

The reason that it has not been used for monitoring is that the survey was cancelled prior to running its complete course. With regard to its lack of use in programme development, however, the reasons are more uncertain and complicated. One possibility is that the survey was not designed to serve directly the developmental research needs of any single programme area, even though broad consultation with the research and health community took place prior to its initiation. Another is that the group which carried out the survey was disbanded shortly after producing its initial report. As a result, there wasn't any systematic follow-through in an attempt to translate results into terms that are programmatically meaningful or to assist programme people in using the findings. In other words, the Canada Health Survey may not have been used for programme development purposes due to the lack of an on-going relationship between the researchers who carried it out and the people responsible for developing programmatic responses in health promotion.

Whatever the reasons, however, it is clear that the results of the survey have been under-utilized from both the point of view of programme development and monitoring of health promotion. Unfortunately, this is not the only example of under-utilization of study results. There are many other studies that have been done in Canada in the recent past where this has also been the case.

Shortage of comparable sub-national data

Although there have been studies of health behaviours at regional or local levels in Canada, where comparisons with other parts of the country or with

Canada as a whole have been possible, such studies have been rare. Thus, health promotion programmers at the sub-national level have not generally had access to results of research which pertain directly to the area for which they are responsible and which could be placed in the context of provincial or national norms. This makes it difficult for programmers to develop health promotion programmes which are appropriate to and useful for their own unique circumstances. There is thus a need to develop strategies for promoting comparability in data collection at all levels in Canada.

Absence of comprehensive long-term planning

To date, much of the research designed to aid in the development of health promotion programmes in Canada at the national level has been carried out on an *ad hoc* basis, in response to the specific requirements of individual programmes. Although there is some merit in such an approach in that the resulting research does tend to meet the needs of those programmes, it would be desirable to be able to have a long-term plan based on a comprehensive assessment of information requirements.

The value of doing so is demonstrated by a recent effort to develop and implement an overall plan for the evaluation and monitoring of Health Promotion Directorate projects. Specifically, because of the requirements for evaluating the Health Promotion Directorate programme as a whole, an Evaluation Framework was produced in early 1984 (Program Evaluation Directorate 1984). One of the requirements of this framework was that the Directorate develop a system to monitor and evaluate its projects. Such a system has in fact been developed and is currently being implemented. Among other things, it requires regular comprehensive assessments of the evaluation and monitoring needs of all Directorate projects. While it is too early to say what its long-term impact will be on the quality and coverage of our monitoring and evaluation efforts, it is quite clear that this process has helped us to obtain a rational overview of our needs and to allocate resources on the basis of rationally established priorities. It is apparent that a similar kind of effort would be beneficial with regard to research for programme development.

Correcting the deficiencies

Given the deficiencies in our use of research for developing health promotion programmes in Canada, what corrective actions might be taken? Possibilities for reducing each of the three major deficiencies will be discussed in turn.

Encouraging use of research

As suggested above, one key reason why health behaviour research has not been used more for programme development is the lack of an ongoing relationship between researchers and programmers. It is not always easy for researchers to work with programme people. Differences in values, world views, backgrounds, training, and time frames sometimes create difficulties. However, there is much to be gained from trying to find ways of working together more effectively. One such way is substantially to involve programme people in the specification of information needs. The value of such an approach has been demonstrated in the development of our National Health Promotion Survey. This survey took over three years to develop—a long time by anyone's standards! But one of the reasons why it took so long is that the survey developers went out of their way to involve programme people at all stages. At the very beginning the latter were asked to indicate in writing specifically what information they hoped to obtain from the survey that would be useful to them in planning their programmes. Their needs were then discussed in a group setting with all researchers and programme people present. As the survey developed, they were given drafts of the instruments to comment on and were interviewed individually about their comments. If their needs could not be satisfied by the survey, it was explained why this was the case. Although this process was painful in some instances for both the researchers and programme people, the outcome has been the creation of a group of programme people who understand the survey, are sympathetic to it, have rapport with the researchers, are eagerly awaiting its results and will participate in their dissemination.

Another way of working with programme people to exploit the programme development potential of existing research is to try to assist them in interpreting and using findings. Typically, research reports are prepared by researchers, for researchers. Too often programmers are simply sent a completed report which may be too technical or too voluminous for them to use effectively. Or they may not even be aware that such reports exist. Some ways of correcting this problem may be to prepare non-technical summaries which suggest programme implications, to hold debriefing sessions when reports are completed, or to arrange for individual conversations between the researchers and the programme people.

One other way of insuring an ongoing working relationship between researchers and programme people is to assign researchers to programme and project teams. Although our Directorate has not uniformly done this, in the instances in which it has occurred it has been found to be profitable from everyone's point of view. It has alerted the researchers to information requirements that have led subsequently to studies and it has made programme people aware of the results of research in a dynamic and useful way.

There are certainly other ways of ensuring good working relations between researchers and programme people but the main point is that it is vitally important that means be found to establish such relations if research is to become more useful for programme development.

Another reason why the results of research are under-utilized for programme development purposes is that the data are not as accessible as they might be. One attempt we have recently made to correct this problem is to publish an inventory of health promotion data sets. The net result is a compilation of descriptions of about 50 Canadian sets on health behaviours in loose leaf form (Rootman and Brown 1985). It has just been distributed to researchers and workers in the health promotion field, so we don't as yet know how large an impact it will have on the utilization of data for programme development purposes, but we are encouraged by the fact that it has been requested not only by researchers but also by programme people. It is our intention to update the inventory and to follow-up to see how it is being used.

Other possibilities for making data more accessible which we are currently discussing include conferences of health promotion data users, development of manuals, and the preparation of a library of health promotion data sets on micro-computer discs.

Promoting comparability

One possibility for promoting comparability of local studies, is to design national studies in such a way as to permit inclusion of local areas. This in fact is the strategy which we have adopted for the National Health Promotion Survey. Specifically, equal sized samples (about 1000 cases) have been drawn in each province and territory in Canada to permit generalization to these jurisdictions as well as to the national level. In addition, the possibility of supplementing the sample for local areas was permitted and at least one community has taken advantage of it.

Another possibility for promoting comparability is to produce guidelines which can be followed by those wishing to carry out local studies. In the National Health Promotion survey for instance, guidelines based on the procedures followed nationally will be produced and made available on request. Similarly, guidelines for student surveys of drug use have been produced in Canada (Smart 1985). Although it is too soon to say whether or not such guidelines will be effective in promoting comparability, there is reason to be hopeful. No doubt, other possibilities for promoting comparability exist as well.

Comprehensive long-term planning

While, as illustrated by the fate of the Canada Health Survey, it is not always possible to execute long-term plans for research, it is nevertheless desirable to do so. Accordingly, we are currently reviewing our internal research needs and, in collaboration with the National Health Research Development Programme which is the major programme for funding research in our Department, will be reviewing the external requirements for health promotion research. We hope that this process will produce an overall plan for developmental research for our Directorate that will reflect the long-term needs of our programme as well as a set of priorities for the country. This is not the only way to do long-term planning for developmental research in the health promotion field, but it is perhaps one that is worth considering.

Conclusion

This chapter has reviewed the Canadian experience in the use of health behaviour research for programme development and monitoring in the health promotion field. In addition to presenting examples of how research has been used for these purposes in Canada, it presented examples of how it has been used for other equally important purposes such as informing people and stimulating action. The chapter also identified three deficiencies in the conduct and use of health behaviour research in Canada—under-utilization, shortage of comparble sub-national data, and absence of long-term planning. Some possible solutions for the latter were then presented.

The suggestions that have been made are by no means the only, or even necessarily the best, ways to redress these deficiencies. However, one recurrent theme emerged—the need for all health professionals in the health promotion field to make an effort to work together and share their unique talents, experiences, and insights if our common objectives are to be addressed. In that sense, the principles suggested herein imply that our fundamental philosophy as health researchers must be consistent with our overall philosophy of health promotion. Our role is to *enable* other health professionals to better achieve the objectives we all share. If we do so effectively we will be more likely to achieve our universal goal of 'health for all by the year 2000'.

References

Canadian Mental Health Association (1984). *Work and well-being: the changing realities of employment*. Canadian Mental Health Association, Toronto.
COGEM, Inc. (1984). *Health education/education sanitaire readership survey*. Health and Welfare Canada, Ottawa.
Collishaw, N. and Myers, G. (1984). Dollar estimates of the consequences of tobacco use in Canada, 1979. *Canadian Journal of Public Health* 75, pp. 192–9.
European Office of World Health Organization (1984). *Health promotion: a discussion document on the concepts and principles*. World Health Organization, Copenhagen.
Garceau, S. (1985). *Alcohol, tobacco and marijuana use and norms among young people in Canada—Year 3*. Health and Welfare, Canada, Ottawa.
Goldfarb Consultants (1981a). *Smoking and non-smoking—a study of Canadians' behaviour and attitudes*. Health and Welfare Canada, Ottawa.

Goldfarb Consultants (1981b). *Anti-smoking pre-test*. Health and Welfare Canada, Ottawa.

Health and Welfare Canada (1983). *Canadian initiatives in smoking and health*. Health and Welfare Canada, Ottawa.

Health and Welfare Canada and Statistics Canada (1981). *The health of Canadians*. Statistics Canada, Ottawa.

Jossa, D. (1985). *Smoking behaviour of Canadians, 1983*. Health and Welfare Canada, Ottawa.

King, A. J. C., Robertson, A., Warren, W. K., and Fuller, K. R. (1984). *Summary report: Canada health knowledge survey, 1982/83*. Health and Welfare Canada, Ottawa.

Lalonde, M. (1974). *A new perspective on the health of Canadians*. Health and Welfare Canada, Ottawa.

McDowell, I. and Praught, E. (1982). On the measurement of happiness. *American Journal of Epidemiology* **116**, 949–58.

Millar, W. J. and Bartlett, J. M. (1985). *The 'time to quit' smoking cessation program: a report on evaluation findings, January 1982 to December 1983*. Health and Welfare Canada, Ottawa.

Millar, W. J. and Van Rensburg, S. (1983). *Tobacco use among students in the Northwest Territories, 1982*. Health and Welfare Canada, Ottawa.

Program Evaluation Directorate (1984). *Health promotion evaluation framework*. Health and Welfare Canada, Ottawa.

Rootman, I. and Brown, D. (1985). *Health promotion research data files*. Health and Welfare Canada and Public Archives Canada, Ottawa.

Smart, R. (1985). *Guidelines for the development of Canadian surveys of alcohol and drug use among students*. Health and Welfare Canada, Ottawa.

Working Group on Alcohol Statistics (1984). *Alcohol in Canada: a national perspective*. Health and Welfare Canada, Ottawa.

18

National health education programmes

JOHN K. DAVIES

Introduction

The past ten years have seen an unprecedented growth in public interest in health and rapid changes in the practice of health education. Throughout this chapter I will refer to health education developments in Scotland, but they do apply also in general terms in many other countries. In the mid-1970s health education was firmly based on the medical model of illness. Priority was given, due to high mortality and morbidity rates, to lung cancer and chronic bronchitis, alcoholism, and dental caries. Health education was seen as a form of secondary prevention which sought to communicate to those 'at risk'. It attempted to inform them of the signs and symptoms of their potential 'illness', so that they could accept the 'at risk' role and go along to a health professional for appropriate treatment. Each campaign was specifically related to an issue, such as smoking, alcohol, dental health, or family planning. Since the mid-1970s a variety of factors have combined, causing a step-by-step process from secondary, through primary prevention of ill-health conditions, through to attempts to promote a positive concept of good health. At the same time health education policies began to shift responsibility for health from the health professional to the individual (*Help Yourself to Health* was the title of a SHEG self-help booklet which epitomized this development). In 1984 SHEG launched a campaign around the slogan—'Be all you can be—go for good health'. Its aim, taking into account Scottish people's life styles, was to speak meaningfully in terms of positive personal development, not just physical health but also of social and mental health. Under the umbrella of this campaign a number of specific issues have subsequently been tackled.

Role of research in health education

The above changes in health education have been reflected in the use made of research. In the 1960s and 1970s interest arose in the role of psychological factors in health-related behaviour (Kasl and Cobb 1966a, 1966b; Mechanic 1968). During this period various theories of health behaviour, based on such social psychological models, were applied to health education practice (Baum *et al*. 1984). Therefore, research at this time tended to concentrate on psychological analyses of individual at-risk behaviours. A good example was the pioneering work carried out at the University of Strathclyde in Glasgow (Jahoda and Cramond 1972; Davies and Stacey 1972; Aitken 1978). These three studies covered the formulation and development of attitudes to alcohol of children from 6 to 17 years. On the basis of the data obtained from these studies, three films with teachers' notes were prepared for schools and youth clubs. This data also helped in the Scottish Health Education Unit's anti-smoking programme which developed the themes of parental exemplar and personal choice. Other research studies had been used extensively in the development of these campaigns and those aimed at adults (McKennell and Thomas 1967; Bynner 1969). Market research companies were used to monitor specific campaigns in an attempt to assess awareness. Epidemiological data, together with sales and production figures of substances such as alcohol and tobacco, were used to define priority areas and identify potential target populations. Various attempts were made to monitor and evaluate a variety of small-scale intervention studies—these tended to be types of 'action research' where the intervening agent was expected to carry out their own research (e.g. feasibility of self-help groups in stopping smoking; development of hospital in-patient education system for coronary rehabilitation; role of health education in health centres; integration of health education materials in secondary schools; patient education about mastectomy; use of pharmacists in health education about smoking; GUS kit (give up smoking) in general practice; role of self-help groups in dysmenorrhoea; and so on). Standard pre-post test evaluations were carried out on some of SHEU's main campaigns (e.g. Henderson 1980; Plant *et al*. 1979).

Barriers to the effective use of health-behaviour research

Health-behaviour research during the 1970s was primarily epidemiologically based, and relied on theories of individual psychology which related to specific risk-behaviours, e.g. smoking, alcohol abuse, unprotected sex. Its use by health educators was of an *ad hoc* nature. There were no on-going surveys of health behaviour—research was applied in an unsophisticated unsystematic way. There were a number of reasons for this state of affairs.

Lack of an established infrastructure

Unlike some other countries, the UK lacked an infrastructure in applied research terms which was readily accessible to health education practitioners. The major Government research organization—the Social Survey Division of the Office of Population Censuses and Surveys (OPCS)—has always had the highest reputation for high quality research work. They have carried out a number of surveys which have been utilized by health educators but there are many conflicting calls on their services from all sectors of Government and public service.

Therefore, although their research surveys have occasionally been repeated over the years, they cannot provide an on-going social survey facility specifically related to the needs of health educators. Their work usually covers Great Britain (Marsh and Matheson 1983) and often England and Wales only (Breeze 1985a); where Scotland is covered within British surveys, samples are not large enough to produce meaningful Scottish data. Often these surveys are interesting but have limited practical use due to the regional variation in behaviour that do exist (see Bostock and Davies 1980; Breeze 1985b). There are two exceptions: first, the General Household Survey. This interdepartmental survey is sponsored by the Central Statistical Office. It is a continuous survey based on a sample of the general population resident in private households in Great Britain and has been running since 1971. One of the five main subject areas it has covered is health. Included in this section since 1972 has been smoking behaviour (now included every two years) and, since 1978, drinking behaviour. Separate (unpublished) data is available for Scotland. This latter data has been used for health education purposes although a great deal of additional work is required to make it useful to practitioners—see Bostock and Davies (1979) and Ledwith (1982). Secondly, there are those surveys which have been carried out by OPCS on specific Scottish samples (e.g. Knight and Wilson 1980; Goddard 1986; Dobbs and Marsh 1985; Dight 1976). There have been difficulties in relating to OPCS before, during, and after surveys as relationships are usually conducted on a formal basis through Government departments, and often practitioners (those who will use the data) are not involved in detailed discussions. A recent exception to this is the DHSS Committee on Research into the Behavioural Aspects of Smoking and Health, which contains health education planners among others and has successfully steered some more recent work (Marsh and Matheson 1983; Dobbs and Marsh 1985). Resulting from this a successful seminar for practitioners was held in Edinburgh by ASH/SHEG on the applicability to health education of the results of these surveys (Crofton *et al*. 1985).

In addition to the work of OPCS, research is normally carried out by market research companies or academic researchers in universities or research institutes. Both these sources of research expertise have been utilized for health behaviour research purposes by health educators but problems have been encountered. Market research companies are in business to make profit, they are expensive and operate on an *ad hoc* basis from project to project. A decision has to be made between the validity of using their methodology and results (with a quick turnover) against the often painstaking approach of university researchers who are more concerned to advance the frontiers of human knowledge often for half a dozen of their peers. An interesting ethical point arises here also—whether academic researchers should succumb to pressures from policy makers or practitioners or should their academic freedom allow them to decide on research priorities. A second problem has arisen when relating to university researchers in that their contracts and work are often short-term, they work from contract to contract. All of these factors have contributed to the lack of a pool of on-going expertise in the area of health behaviour research applicable to health education practice.

Problem of obtaining appropriate research funding sources

Health education practitioners face the problem that apart from the small funds allocated to research by agencies such as SHEG and the Health Education Council, the larger health research funding bodies are still geared to support clinical and health service delivery research. Often health behaviour research of use to applied fields, such as health education, cannot attract funding or has extreme difficulty in receiving funding from both Government sources and research foundations (McQueen 1986). Practitioners, funders, and researchers would agree that we should strive for 'scientific' respectability but this has to be balanced against the problems of research not being used because it is practically inappropriate.

Concentration on communication parameters

Due to heavy reliance in the past by health educators on social psychological models, much research has concentrated on communication parameters related to communication of the health message. This research has included the assessment of underlying beliefs, attitudes, knowledge, and sometimes behavioural intentions. Rarely has research concentrated in such depth on health behaviour.

Governmental policy changes affecting health education programmes

These changes can occur in a 'negative' sense when the results of research commissioned on health behaviour related to family planning practices cannot be applied in actual campaigns due to political, religious, or moral pressures. In a 'positive' sense these changes can cause health education agencies to change tack in the short-term and concentrate on 'new' behaviours, such as illegal drug use and behaviour related to AIDS. In the latter case quick action is needed and this can affect the health behaviour research being done or needing to be done.

Timescales

Often the research findings from health behaviour research are needed quickly to aid immediate decision-making. The results of long-term cohort studies or trials cannot be awaited. Therefore, the results of longer-term research, although of obvious interest and relevance, cannot be usefully applied in the short term. For example, a longer-term piece of research into the use of SHEG's *Book of the Child* has been received at a time when the resources to re-edit were not available (MacAskill *et al.* 1986). These constantly changing priorities can make for complex situations, not understood by researchers.

Campaign objectives

Sometimes there may be a range of objectives expected from specific health education campaigns by different agencies. In these situations it may be difficult for research to be applied to meet the needs of all parties. For example, these objectives could be 'political' or local versus national objectives, or medical versus educational/behavioural objectives.

Usefulness of health behaviour research

Before considering the application of health behaviour research, national health education programmes need research work classified in the following subdivisions: (*a*) conceptual development, i.e. the multi-disciplinary exploration of concepts underlying health educative efforts; (*b*) effective policy and the provisions of services, i.e. the role and numbers of health education specialists related to other health personnel; (*c*) methodological issues, i.e. the development of more appropriate measures of health-related behaviour; and (*d*) the evaluation of effectiveness and efficiency in health education practice. The latter area has been the most prolific and relevant area to the application of health behaviour research. In this context research is seen as a disciplined form of enquiry encapsulating research, evaluation, and information/intelligence gathering.

Since the late 1970s SHEG has adopted a more systematic use of health-related behaviour research in its national health education planning. Before giving detailed examples of the application of this research, I should identify the major research subdivisions as follows:

1. Basic.
2. Strategic.
3. Developmental.
4. Process.
5. Outcome

Basic research

This can be used to set priorities, define appropriate target groups, and provide the information necessary for the design of effective health education programmes (Davies 1979). Basic research can set baselines enabling the clear formulation of realistic objectives. This research is obtained from a variety of published and unpublished sources. For example the survey of *Scottish Drinking Habits* (Dight 1976) was commissioned by SHEU through OPCS and used to design the Unit's alcohol strategy in the latter half of the 1970s. This was the first national survey carried out anywhere in Great Britain into the drinking behaviour and attitudes of the adult population. This research highlighted for the unit (SHEU) the major target group of young (18–30-year-old) male manual workers as the group most at risk to alcohol abuse. It was found that 3 per cent of the Scottish adult population drank 30 per cent of the total alcohol consumed. Therefore SHEU produced a campaign based on a series of alcohol education 'fillers' aimed at TV and cinema which communicated directly to the above target group and attacked many of the Scottish myths related to alcohol (such as manliness, maturity, etc.) which were so strongly identified in Dight and other previous work. The Scottish Drinking Habits report acted as a basis for further development of SHEG's alcohol programme—based around young alcoholic testimonials— and acted as a basis for the self-monitoring work of the late 1970s/early 1980s. Another example, this time in the area of sexual relations, was the work in the late 1970s related to family planning behaviour. The unit identified two target groups from previous basic research (themes in family planning-basic research): married women who had achieved desired family size, and young unmarried girls. Work was commissioned into the social and psychological correlates of contraceptive risk-taking and discontinuation (McGlew and Harcus 1979). This acted as the basis of SHEU's family planning campaign in the late 1970s. Further work was commissioned on contraceptive behaviour in the early development of the SHEG 'Options' campaign aimed at young people (Leathar and Bostock 1982). Similar work has been used in the development of specific health education campaigns and strategies—dental health campaigns (Todd and Dodd 1985); dental health, behaviour, and attitudes among young people (Leathar and Hastings 1982); dissemination of the *Book of the Child* (Childhood 5–10: parental experience—MacAskill and MacDonald 1982); food hygiene in shops campaign (*Consumer Attitudes towards Food Poisoning*—Hastings 1980); smoking campaigns (Marsh and Matheson 1983; Dobbs and Marsh 1985); NOP smoking habits; System Three Young People; fit for life positive health campaign; NOP hobbies and holidays, survey on leisure activities; fitness and health concepts—Eadie and Leathar 1986; national fitness survey; SHEG's sensible drinking strategy (drinking environment—attitudes to licensing in Scotland—Goddard 1986).

The combination of primary and secondary data on social and environmental indicators is combined with professional views and consumer views to identify needs and priorities for health education.

Strategic research

In combination with the information obtained from the basic research findings, SHEG commissions problem-definition research using detailed studies of levels of knowledge, attitudes, and beliefs. This concept-testing helps decision-making as to the most appropriate health education strategy to be adopted. For example, in relation to smoking, evidence has suggested that while working class groups in Scotland are aware of the health arguments against smoking, reinforcing this awareness alone is not productive and may be counter-productive; the means of solving their anxiety must be provided within any health strategy (Leathar 1980b). As Leathar states, based on SHEG funded research, '. . . promoting positive images of non-smoking, and reinforcing emotional values associated with it, is more likely to provide the appropriate emotional context for people to be susceptible to other more direct, more interpersonal sources of influence (such as opinion leaders, peer groups, and counsel groups) rather than the alternative strategy that reinforces negative factors that people are aware of—but choose to ignore because the information fails to fit in with their existing values.' Leathar goes on to give two examples of such strategic research: i.e. whether the problem being addressed is available to mass media or is symptomatic of some under-lying problem (Leathar 1980a; Leathar and Bostock 1981).

Developmental research

This applies to the creative development of health education programmes by means of testing the communication variables and comprehension of the materials to be used. This work is usually, although not exclusively, done for SHEG by its funded research unit at Strathclyde University—the Advertising Research Unit. Recent work has been carried out, for example, on alcohol television commercials, a booklet produced on healthy nutrition, a drugs magazine insert, a television commercial on smoking, mental health campaign materials, whooping cough advertisements, and a booklet on travellers' health. Each of these pieces of research have been used in fine tuning of the materials involved.

Intervention research

This research consists of practical experiments where specific population sub-groups are identified for health education input. Health education is initiated in this practical setting, is monitored and modified according to the relevant feedback received. Recent examples have included the Glasgow 2000 Anti-smoking initiative which is attempting to make Glasgow a non-smoking city by the year 2000 (Inglis and Davies 1985); development of social learning materials for mentally handicapped young people (McEwan and Snow 1985); dissemination of pre-retirement materials (Shakespeare and Harrison 1985); smoking and schoolchildren (Hoffman Research 1985); self-help methods among problem drinkers (Robertson and Plant 1985); and DRAMS (Drinking Reasonably and Moderately with Self Control)—controlled drinking in general practice. Each of these projects involve the study of aspects of health-related behaviour. There is insufficient opportunity to review the application of this research in each individual project. As an example I propose to discuss the development of DRAMS and a related project—'So you want to cut down your drinking'. Both projects involve the use of self-help manuals designed as early intervention for people with drink problems. Extensive evidence (Heather and Robertson 1983) has shown that for many problem drinkers, especially young people at early stages, advice to control their drinking is often more successful than advising total abstinence. In 1983 Heather and Robertson, with support from SHEG, produced a self-help manual in an experimental version entitled '*so you want to cut down your drinking*'. This manual was advertised through the Scottish national and local press; 785 people responded and were given either this manual or a simpler, non-interactive information booklet. It is not possible to give full details of this research here (see Heather, Whitton and Robertson 1985; Heather *et al*. 1986). The researchers found that the greater mean reduction in weekly consumption shown by the manual group after six months was statistically significant when a sub-group who had sought specialist treatment were excluded from the analysis. The results of this research encouraged SHEG to proceed in the production of a published version of the manual which was made available in late 1985. Changes had been made in the content and design of the manual arising from the research. Further research is planned to compare this manual with simple advice and group therapy methods. In addition to the production of this manual, SHEG have developed the related materials for DRAMS with Heather and Robertson. Dight (1976) found that young heavy drinkers were likely to suffer injuries or illness related to their drinking which will cause them to consult their general practitioner. Evidence showed that they would consult their GP three or four times more frequently than average patients. This should offer opportunities to the GP to advise these patients on their drinking but without any supportive advice material many GPs were reluctant to become involved in protracted and probably unsuccessful counselling. Experience on the GUS (give up smoking) kit, which was developed from successful research by Russell *et al* (1979) and shown to be successful in practice (Jamrozik *et al*. 1984), acted as a model for DRAMS. Underlying both these approaches is the assumption that opportunities will arise naturally in the course of the consultation with the GP to discuss drinking and smoking—referred to as 'opportunistic health promotion' (Stott and Davis 1979). It does require the doctor to take the initiative. DRAMS provided the GP with a pack of supportive material, including a self-help guide and diary.

The scheme was piloted in the Highlands and Islands of Scotland (Glen, Hendry and Milton 1986). We are awaiting the results of a controlled trial of DRAMS in the Tayside Region by a team at Dundee University Medical School.

Evaluative research

This makes a judgement about a health education activity. The conventional approach uses a pre–post test methodology. But large-scale evaluations produce many problems because long-term changes in a population's health may not be evident for some time and may not even be related to the specific health education input under investigation. The evaluation of one-off isolated campaigns have tended to give a limited understanding of health-education interventions. Evaluations can only measure short-term changes for practical reasons. Methodologically they face many problems because the situation under consideration is not as clear-cut as in a laboratory, we cannot hold all the variables constant, or repeat the intervention. Control groups are difficult to establish satisfactorily. As mentioned in the early part of this chapter SHEG has attempted 'traditional' evaluation strategies and found them of limited use. In relation to its mass media programmes SHEG has concentrated since the late 1970s on a different style of evaluation. This involves two stages: the monitoring of long-term trends, and the assessment of the communication parameters within the Scottish population, related to specific campaigns. SHEG has not adopted the conventional approach to evaluation because:

1. It assumes a direct model of effectiveness whereas SHEG's campaigns promote change indirectly. SHEG's campaigns do not have the objective of *directly* inducing behaviour change among large groups of the population. They have three basic objectives: (*a*) to create awareness and knowledge of specific health issues; (*b*) to maintain this awareness in the light of other counter-influences; and (*c*) indirectly to change attitudes and behaviour by promoting the appropriate context in which more direct sources of influence can operate (whether primary care, school or self help support group).
2. Any changes eventually occurring will happen in the longer term.
3. Any short-term changes cannot be picked up by the conventional pre–post methods since they are not sensitive to fine variations.

Recent evaluations of this sort have been carried out on the Group's sponsoring of the Scottish Football Cup, Walkaboutabit, Drugs Campaigns, and Dental Health Campaigns (Schou 1986). To aid the longer-term monitoring of effects SHEG has commissioned a major health tracking study to be carried out, in the first instance, twice a year for the next three years.

This is particularly important in helping to assess the more innovative life style oriented campaigns such as 'be all you can be'.

Future developments

In giving impetus to the Chief Scientist Office (SHHD) in Scotland (Davies 1978), in the establishment of the Working Party on Behavioural Research Priorities (SHHD 1981), and through its support to the Research Unit in Health and Behavioural Change (RUHBC) at the University of Edinburgh, SHEG realized the need to concentrate effort on the study of health-behavioural measures to supplement its past concentration on communication measures. Such behavioural measures would be used to monitor the health behaviour of the Scottish people. For this reason SHEG has been discussing for some time the development of a 'life style and health monitoring programme' with the RUHBC. Significant parts of this programme are now underway: health behaviour in schoolchildren—funded by SHEG as part of its role as a WHO Collaborating Centre; life style and health survey of 18–44-year-olds—funded by SHEG; health behaviour in 45–59-year-olds—funded by the Health Services Research Committee of the Central Statistical Office; and health behaviour of the elderly—being processed with the Centres for Ageing. Once fully underway this programme would provide a broader behavioural base for health-education activities in Scotland. It would assist in monitoring the long-term cumulative effects of health-education activities and help with more sophisticated targetting since, having identified the behavioural risk factors, research is needed to determine whether changing this behaviour will have any effect in preventing or treating the illness. This health-behaviour monitoring programme will identify patterns of behaviour, whether these types of behaviour cluster together, and whether factors exist which can predict behaviour change. This information will help not only in the development of more sophisticated health education interventions but also aid monitoring and evaluation.

Conclusions

1. Further research is needed into health-related behaviours and how such behaviours change over time. To date most research in this area is illness-oriented and concerned with single health behaviours. In Target 32 of WHO European Strategy of Health for All by 2000 (WHO 1985a) they identify the need for a better understanding of the influence of life style on health behaviour. Emphasis must be placed on the development of more sophisticated measures of the variables involved in health behaviour.
2. Definitional problems exist throughout the health-behaviour literature. Attempts should be made at international level to obtain agreement on

the basic definitions, particularly related to terms such as illness behaviour, and protective and preventive health behaviour.
3. More resources in terms of appropriate training of researchers with associated career structures should be established.
4. There is a need for more interdisciplinary co-operation in the field of health-related behaviour (see WHO 1986). This should concentrate specifically on linking the major medical and behavioural spheres in relation to funding (Davies and Mitchell 1986).
5. Research tends to concentrate at single programme level in health education. Efforts being made with National Health Tracking Studies and Lifestyle and Health Monitoring Studies in Scotland should be replicated in other countries.
6. At local level there is a lack of relevant data on health behaviour. The US 'Patch' system should be adopted more widely in other countries (i.e. Centers for Disease Control jointly funds with state authorities opportunities for local people to examine their own health problems and develop appropriate strategies).

An academically based unit such as RUHBC, working closely with a national health education agency such as SHEG, acts as a model for adoption in other countries in order to develop further the application of research in health behaviour to health-education practice.

References

Aitken, P. P. (1978). *Ten-to-fourteen-year-olds and alcohol. A developmental study in the central region of Scotland*. HMSO, Edinburgh.

Baum, A., Taylor, S. E. and Singer, J. E. (1984). *Handbook of psychology and health*, Vol. IV—*Social psychologicl aspects of health*. L. Erlbaum Associates, Hillsdale, N.J.

Bostock, Y. and Davies, J. K. (1979). Recent changes in the prevalence of cigarette smoking in Scotland. *Health Bulletin, Edinburgh* **37**, 260–7.

Bostock, Y. and Davies, J. K. (1980). Recent changes in the prevalence of cigarette smoking in Scotland compared with trends in England and Wales. *Health Trends, London* **12**, 41–4.

Breeze, E. (1985a). *Women and drinking*. HMSO, London.

Breeze, E. (1985b). *Differences in drinking patterns between selected regions*. HMSO, London.

Bynner, J. (1969). *The young smoker*. HMSO, London.

Crofton, J., Hillhouse, A., and Ramsay, I. (1985). A report of a seminar held to discuss the implications for health education and research of recent OPCS surveys on smoking. ASH, SHEG, Chest Heart and Stroke Association, Edinburgh.

Davies, J. B. and Stacey, B. (1972). *Teenagers and alcohol. A developmental study in Glasgow*. HMSO, London.

Davies, J. K. (1978). A discussion paper on health education research for the Health

Services Research Committee of the Chief Scientist Office. SHHD, Edinburgh (unpublished).

Davies, J. K. (1979). Assessing research priorities for health education at national level. Paper presented to the 10th World Conference on Health Education, London.

Davies, J. K. and Mitchell, S. C. (1986). A discussion paper on health education funding for the Common Services Agency Management Committee, Edinburgh (unpublished).

Dight, S. E. (1976). *Scottish drinking habits*. HMSO, London.

Dobbs, J. and Marsh, A. (1985). *Smoking among secondary schoolchildren in 1984*. HMSO, London.

Eadie, D. R. and Leathar, D. S. (1986). *The concepts of fitness and health: an exploratory study*. University of Strathclyde, Glasgow.

Glen, I., Hendry, J., and Milton, A. (1986). DRAMS. A pilot study of controlled drinking in individuals with alcohol abuse presenting to general practitioners in the Highlands and Islands of Scotland.

Goddard, E. (1986). *Drinking and attitudes to licensing in Scotland*. HMSO, London.

Hastings, G. B. (1980). *Consumer attitudes towards food poisoning*. University of Strathclyde, Glasgow.

Heather, N. and Robertson, I. (1983). *Controlled drinking*. Methuen, London.

Heather, N., Whitton, B., and Robertson, I. (1985). *Evaluation of a self help manual for media recruited problem drinkers*.

Heather, N., Robertson, I., MacPherson, B., Allsop, S. and Fulton, A. (1986). *Effectiveness of a controlled drinking self-help manual: one year follow-up results*. Addictive Behaviours Research Group, University of Dundee.

Henderson, R. S. (1980). *A report for the SHEU as a result of smoking in pregnancy programme evaluation over a 5-year period 1975–1980*. Strathclyde Area Survey; University of Strathclyde, Glasgow.

Hoffman Research (1985). *School Kids against Smoking*. Aberdeen.

Inglis, V. and Davies, J. K. (1985). Smoking in Glasgow: a report on the Glasgow 2000 project baseline survey. *Health Bulletin, Edinburgh* **43**, 4–12.

Jahoda, G. and Cramond, J. (1972). *Children and alcohol. A developmental study in Glasgow*. HMSO, London.

Jamrozik, K. *et al*. (1984). Controlled trial of three different anti-smoking interventions in general practice. *British Medical Journal* **286**, 445–53.

Kasl, S. V. and Cobb, S. (1966a). Health behaviour, illness behaviour and sick role behaviour. I. Health and illness behaviour. *Archives of Environmental Health* **12**, 246–66.

Kasl, S. V. and Cobb, S. (1966b). Health behaviour, illness behaviour and sick role behaviour. II. Sick role behaviour. *Archives of Environmental Health* **12**, 531–41.

Knight, I. and Wilson, P. (1980). *Scottish Licensing Laws*. HMSO, London.

Leathar, D. S. (1980a). Smoking amongst student nurses. *Nursing Times*. April, 589–90.

Leathar, D. S. (1980b). Defence inducing advertising. In *Taking stock: what have we learnt and where are we going?* Proceedings of the E.S.O.M.A.R. Conference, Monte Carlo, Sept. pp. 153–73.

Leathar, D. S. (1981). The use of mass media health education campaigns in Scotland. *Journal of the Institute of Health Education* **19**, No. 4.

Leathar, D. S. and Bostock, Y. (1981). The role of mass media advertising campaign in influencing attitudes towards contraception among 16–20 year olds. In *Health education and the media* (eds. D. S. Leathar, G. B. Hastings and J. K. Davies). Pergamon Press, Oxford.

Leathar, D. S. and Bostock, Y. (1982). Attitudes towards contraception among young people. SHEG Occasional Paper, Edinburgh.

Leathar, D. S. and Hastings, G. B. (1982). *Dental care, behaviour and attitudes among young people*. University of Strathclyde, Glasgow.

Ledwith, F. (1982). Smoking trends in Scotland since 1972—conventional wisdom is challenged. *Scottish Medicine* **2**, 16–17.

MacAskill, S. and MacDonald, M. B. (1982). *Childhood 5–10. An exploratory study of parental experience*. University of Strathclyde, Glasgow.

MacAskill, S., MacDonald, M. B., and Leathar, D. S. (1986). *Evaluation of the book of the child*. University of Strathclyde, Glasgow.

Marsh, A. and Matheson, J. (1983). *Smoking attitudes and behaviour*. HMSO, London.

McEwan, C. and Snow, D. (1985). Forth Valley health education project for the mentally handicapped. Paper presented at the 7th World Congress of the International Association for the Scientific Study of Mental Deficiency, New Delhi.

McGlew, T. and Harcus, D. (1979). Rationality and Risk-Taking: a study of family planning practice in marriage. University of Edinburgh.

McKennell, A. C. and Thomas, R. K. (1967). Adults' and adolescents' smoking habits and attitudes. Government Social Survey, London.

McQueen, D. V. (1986). Personal Communication.

Mechanic, D. (1968). *Medical Sociology*. Free Press, New York.

NOP Market Research Ltd. Smoking Habits. (Ongoing).

NOP Market Research Ltd. (1985). A syndicated survey on leisure activities.

NOP Market Research Ltd. (1985). Hobbies and holidays.

Plant, M., Pirie, F., and Kreitman, N. (1979). Evaluation of the SHEU's 1976 campaign on alcoholism. *Social Psychiatry* **14**, 11–24.

Robertson, I. and Plant, M. (1985). Self help methods among problem drinkers. Research Proposal.

Russell, M. A. H. *et al*. (1979). Effect of general practitioners' advice against smoking. *British Medical Journal* **4**, 231–5.

Schou, L. (1986). Evaluation of a national dental health campaign in Scotland. *Community Dentistry and Oral Epidemiology*. (In press).

Scottish Home and Health Department (1981). Report of the Working Party on Behavioural Research Priorities. Chief Scientist Office, Edinburgh.

Shakespeare, P. and Harrison, R. (1985). *Interim report on the dissemination of pre-retirement materials in the community*. Open University, Milton Keynes.

Stott, N. C. H. and Davis, R. H. (1979). The exceptional potential to each primary care consultation. *Journal of the Royal College of General Practitioners* **29**, 201–205.

Todd, J. E. and Dodd, T. (1985). *Children's dental health in the U.K. 1983*. HMSO, London.

World Health Organization, European Office (1985a). *Targets for health for all. Targets in support of the European Regional Strategy for health for all.* Copenhagen.

World Health Organization, European Office (1985b). *Research in health promotion: priorities, strategies, barriers.* Report of a joint WHO/SHEG Workshop, Copenhagen.

SECTION F

Discussion papers on a new agenda for research in health behaviour

19

New perspectives for research in health behaviour

ILONA KICKBUSCH

Within a health promotion approach, it becomes necessary to see health-related and health-directed practices as an expression of social and cultural patterns. Health promotion aims at developing individual competence to reorient actions within this pattern, at transcending the pattern or, through environmental intervention, at reorienting the pattern towards health.

Since health promotion does not aim at changing personalities but at enabling positive health practices, we need to consider specific contexts in which individuals or groups tend to behave in a certain way (in pubs, under stress, while driving a car) and provide suggestions and opportunities on how these 'social situations' could be restructured to encourage new patterns of behaviour. Within psychology, this has been termed 'the grammar of social situations'; within anthropology, it would refer mainly to boundaries and rituals. At its best, health promotion would be part of an open social process which gradually changes values in society, with relevant groups acting as agents of change rather than a 'closed' approach of prescription and prohibition from above. Of course, such redefinitions of contextual behaviour may often clash with values which are more important than health to the group concerned and cannot escape a highly normative stance.

But redefinitions of norms and rituals are continually being produced and developed by various sectors of society. Religion, the media, and industry play a central role, as in the strategy of the cigarette industry to increase sales in the Third World or the opposition to family planning by some religious and political leaders.

The place we give to health in our lives, as compared with other concerns, may differ from person to person; it differs at various stages of the life cycle. The place of health may differ from society to society, and it is both socio-economic and cultural factors which determine this difference.

Health cultures

Approaching the person–environment interaction in cultural terms allows us to understand how individuals structure reality, what meanings they attach to certain actions and practices, what patterns of meaning and practices exist, how they are distributed within a society, and how boundaries are drawn between groups. The identification of patterns allows us to reflect the order a group of people or a society have given the individual environment interaction.

The investigations of the cultural dimension of health would give particular emphasis to three notions.

1. *The personal interpretations that help individuals to adapt to everyday experiences of health and illness.* A perspective on culture allows us to challenge the notion that developed societies live only according to cognitive rules. People have not only needs but also dreams and desires. Dreams can lead actions as much as can dire necessity. To put it in simple terms: your dream of looking or being like Lauren Bacall or Humphrey Bogart will be one of the elements which make you reach for a cigarette and hold it in a certain way. The dream of what constitutes the good life will influence your way of coping with reality. Dreams keep people alive and they drive them to their death. They can be individual or collective. Many other societies acknowledge the reality of dreams and cannot understand the exclusion of this other world from Western culture.

2. *The role of rituals.* Boundaries and rituals constitute an order within societies which makes behaviour within a certain context predictable and gives security for everyday actions. Social change brings with it the break-down of this predictability, and periods of transition in society require special attention in relation to their health consequences. On an individual level, most societies have developed rituals to deal with both positive and difficult life transitions, such as puberty or death. Developed societies tend to offer professional rituals for such social events rather than community-based rituals. New community-based rituals are slowly being developed, in self-help groups for example, to fill the gap.

3. *The boundaries between health systems and the order and rules that maintain boundaries.* Analysis along these lines would help to clarify which group or groups have the power to define what is accepted as normal in terms of health and illness, and at what points the boundaries of the acceptable are extended due to strong pressure or social change. The respective health worlds or health cultures reflect the power structure within health and the structure of communication within each health world. These elements allow us to define the dominant approach to health within a society or towards a specific group and to analyse what level of medicalization or professionalization has been reached.

Patterns of health practices

Health promotion looks at general behaviour in the context of health and at specific health behaviour in its wider social context. People's lives are their health, but health is not their reason for living. The value attached to health differs greatly between and within societies. Research into health behaviour, health practices, and health actions has only just begun to identify positive and negative health practices and to relate them to the individual's position in the social structure and the way of life in a society. Some existing research could be reinterpreted with this view in mind.

It is useful to identify two types of health behaviour:

- health-directed practices which are consciously undertaken to maintain health or reduce illness;
- health-related practices which are part of everyday life and either directly or indirectly influence a person's health status.

Health-related practices are practically impossible to isolate from the general life style of a society or cultural group. This tendency to isolate health-related practices, such as smoking, has led to risk factor programmes that have focused on the direct and isolated relationship between a certain practice and its health outcome, i.e. smoking and heart disease, while neglecting the position of a person in society. This position is important in two ways: (*a*) in relation to socio-economic and demographic variables such as poverty, gender, education, or age, which are in themselves interrelated in structured ways; and (*b*) in relation to the meaning attached to certain practices in everyday life within the context of one's reference group.

In most investigations of lay health and illness behaviour, these subjects have been defined predominantly in terms of the use of professional services. Even the studies that have investigated the subject of self-care may define the concept narrowly as the use of herbal or chemical substances and in terms of a dichotomy—as behaviour alternative to contacting professional care-givers. Such a limited concept of self-care behaviour may exclude some of its most beneficial forms, such as stress containment or responses to illness, which are directed towards the cause rather than the alleviation of symptoms.

It is known from those few investigations that have reviewed the full range of self-care from the individual's perspective, that the range of self-care is exceedingly wide. Health-protective behaviour may include alterations in diet, smoking or use of alcohol, obtaining fresh air or exercise, relaxation techniques, or changing daily routines. Forms of social interaction have been reported as both health maintenance and symptom-response self-care.

Risk behaviour and coping: a social approach to health-behaviour research

The cutting edge between concepts of risk behaviour and concepts of coping can be illustrated as follows: in order to get through everyday life, many people endanger their health and are constantly exposed to health threats which are beyond their immediate control. They have to develop modes of coping, i.e. modes of managing demands from both external and internal sources.

People face health risks every day. Risk behaviour is a form of coping, but it is usually understood in a narrow sense as 'a behaviour leading to a risk of losing one's health'. The phrase has gained particular prominence within epidemiological research in relation to risk factors such as smoking, cholesterol, and high blood pressure. The concept of epidemiological risk has ruled the planning of health care over the years. Risk factors have been defined when the research has revealed a relationship between a disease and some single factor. While in many cases it has not been possible to prove a causal relationship, it has been possible in some, as in the relationship of smoking to several diseases. The notion of 'health risk' has been expanded gradually by the medical system. For example, in the ever-increasing intervention of medicine in childbirth, women have consistently lost part of their freedom to opt for a particular type of behaviour and/or treatment. Studies of alternative services show that one of the special attractions of those services for the public is that they have adopted a different concept of risk, in that the persons concerned are involved in the decision-making process and are allowed to make the final choice. Risk factors have served as the basis for health education, which has been planned from the angle of one single risk factor (or, more rarely, several single factors at the same time). This approach has been criticized heavily because it splits up behaviours and is based on single habits, it explains only a small percentage of morbidity, and it does not include the assessment of risk by the population itself.

Theoretical and educational models often assume that human behaviour is a relatively rational striving towards the best possible solutions from the health point of view. We are increasingly being faced with the fact that it is difficult to create general models of the conformities of human behaviour. People do not necessarily rationalize their behaviour according to one single value. Marketing research builds on the values of fantasies and dreams, hopes and desires, not on rational guidelines for behaviour.

The context of risk behaviour

Risk behaviour may constitute a way in which the individual can deal with conflicts that arise in everyday life and regain the physical and psychological ability to face up to them again. The risks are taken personally, with an eye to individual benefit, not to the degree of social acceptance or rejection they may provoke. Often such behaviour patterns are highly acceptable within a culture and are promoted by the mass media, advertising, and traditions. 'You need a drink', 'take a pill', 'have a cigarette', etc., are phrases suggesting that coping with conflict situations is a matter of conformity. Attempts to encourage individuals to adopt positive coping styles must allow for the fact that their present behaviour is not merely a matter of free choice; it may more often be a desperate reaction in an attempt to find a way to deal with individual problems as well as the problems of society.

In industrialized countries, the increasing number of recognized health hazards has made it difficult to perceive their reality and extent. Health risks are nowadays discussed daily, and they seem constantly to increase in amount. There is little research on how people experience risks posed to their health and how much control they feel they have over them. Environmental risk, the threat of war and the fear of unemployment are risks viewed quite differently by professionals, decision-makers, and members of the public. Health is often a receding factor compared with price policy, agricultural policy, or employment policy. Policy decisions which increase health risks are often consciously made from a purely economic perspective. The discrepancy is even greater for developing countries where economic development is seen as a guarantee for better health.

Risk behaviour plays a major role in establishing an identity and in testing the control the individual has over the environment and self; this aspect of risk behaviour is important in understanding why some young people adopt patterns of behaviour that involve risks for their health; only too often such patterns are merely dubbed 'irresponsible' rather than being considered in the context of a period of transition from one stage of life to another. Perhaps social, emotional, and physical well-being are not always compatible.

Feelings of powerlessness are a major factor in understanding risk behaviour. Any decision on how to act or react in a social situation is determined by what risks are considered acceptable, but acceptability is not always subject to individual control.

Many 'unhealthy choices', as currently defined, must be viewed in their wider social context—the social conditions under which health-damaging 'choices' occurs reflect efforts at stress management and coping, a desire to conform to peer group norms, or a minimal expression of power in the context of lives characterized by isolation, alienation, or excessive strain. We must ask if some risk reduction campaigns and screening programmes have a negative impact on health by increasing fear of cancer and of some of the other so-called 'killer diseases'. We need to expand our knowledge base to include assessments of the social and psychological consequences of the increased awareness of risk factors and prevention approaches.

Health education efforts are often most effective when recipients feel at risk of damage or need to prevent something they wish to avoid. We need to ask if there are 'tipping points' beyond which individuals experience everything they do as so 'risky' that it is best to ignore all such advice—or even take up especially hazardous activities of behaviour. The experience of probable death from nuclear war, for example, must be explored as a factor which undermines attempts to motivate people to reduce ordinary risks in everyday life.

The context of coping

If we move coping into a social context, we can see that no given pattern of coping works in the same way in all circumstances. But we can at the same time trace patterns of coping for classes of people and classes of contexts. We can also show that, in certain contexts, certain coping resources and coping skills have made all the difference. Health promotion therefore seeks to open coping options to both individuals and groups.

Risk behaviour involves both coping styles and options for coping. If it is the cultural pattern learned from early life that one takes a drink after work to relax or offers a cigarette in order to get to know somebody, the health effects of this behaviour will not be important in the decision. Coping takes on a specific meaning when seen first as a pattern learned within a culture. We can distinguish between coping mechanisms which influence health:

- general coping styles which are cultural in origin and can have positive or negative health effects on health status;
- coping styles which are consciously undertaken to promote health and well-being, and to cope with illness.

We must stress the relational aspect of coping, its role as a component of a larger culture and society. The individual learns to employ culturally constituted coping mechanisms which influence not only behaviour but also feelings along the lines of cultural patterns and codes. This applies not only to normal behaviour but also holds true for deviant behaviour. Reactions which are termed irrational by professionals often show a clear meaning when defined in a cultural context.

Coping processes are in no way always appraised consciously. The more they are linked to the strains of everyday life rather than specific events, the more they will be coped with routinely or by certain rituals. The process merges the individual coping traits, the cultural coping styles and the society's barriers and reinforcements.

Health-behaviour research of a new type

Health promotion takes a different view of people and their problems; it credits them with an awareness and will to influence the situation. Traditional public health ranks risks according to mortality statistics. Health promotion which starts from the people's definition of needs would concentrate especially on those factors the people see as a threat to their everyday well-being.

The level of daily well-being free from pain, anxiety, and depression would be measured and a high value would be placed on subjectively perceived health. Within a health-promotion approach, health potential is a central principle of evaluation. We need to research systematically the effects of nurturing and caring on well-being as on conventional morbidity and mortality outcomes. We also need to research how informal care-giving is performed in all societies in ways which address explicitly the sex of both care-givers and receivers, and the implications of gender for both the delivery and receipt of health-promoting activities. In the poor countries of the world, providing basic goods for a better quality of life and avoiding early death are still fundamental preoccupations. In developed societies, days of impaired well-being measured within a population with a similar life expectancy give a clearer indication of actual health than the mortality indicators normally applied.

If we knew more about the distribution of these experiences of impaired well-being, we might alter our perception of the relative importance of the so-called killer diseases such as cancer and heart disease. A new epidemiology of everyday health actions might suggest new priorities for allocating resources for preventive care and supportive services. In the framework of this new epidemiology, 'healthy life-styles' would no longer focus on individual 'risk factor reduction' but on new definitions of significant health actions and health potential.

20

The need for new social policy perspectives in health-behaviour research

PIERPAOLO DONATI

The issue and a general framework

Social policy perspectives on health behaviour are frequently mentioned but hardly ever focused upon. Even the chapters presented in this book deal with social policy issues in a superficial way. It is therefore necessary to find a general framework which can elucidate the complex interrelationships between social policy and health behaviour.

The definition of social policy is problematic: It can be defined as that policy which supports weak social groups or alternatively as the system of actions of a society which affects the whole population. The definition of social policy to be adopted here relates to the general regulation of society in terms of equality (or equity). It is taken to imply fair participation for everyone in the distribution of resources and consequently to a fair distribution of health (Donati 1985).

In this definition society treats health not only as a physical and psychic resource but also as a generalized symbolic medium of interchange which governs the relations among all the societal subsystems such as the family, workplace, educational system, and political subsystem (Donati 1983a). In other words, we have to adopt a relational conception of health (Donati 1983b) in which health and health behaviour are equivalent to healthy social relations in everyday life.

In the perspective of social policy, health behaviour is primarily an issue of societal control and regulation from top down: from welfare state apparatuses to subcultures. International research clearly shows that social policies conceived in this way may have little effect on health behaviour. The symbolic codes and the administrative procedures used by the welfare state are inadequate in relation to everyday life subcultures.

As well as cultural factors there are structural factors which constitute barriers between welfare state apparatuses and health subcultures. These barriers arise from the political and economic limitations of the present welfare state (Donati 1984). Its corporatist structure and fiscal crisis reduce the changes of achieving a preventive health system and the implementation of the programmes of primary care recommended by WHO. This is clear from examination of social policy measures as indicated by the composition of public expenditure in the health sector. These leave little room for the implementation of primary extramural services to foster health subcultures in the community. Also these health subcultures which need socio-cultural and political legitimation are not recognized by the state as primary components of societal action.

A redefinition of social policy aimed at promoting health behaviour through a major involvement of health subcultures should try to change these barriers into resources for the development of non-state social policies. Non-state social policies are seen as being those not-for-profit initiatives which can be self managed by the people through local initiatives, and legitimized and supported financially by local authorities.

This general scheme highlights a number of, as yet, unanswered questions. What kind of concepts of health do policy makers have and how do these relate to the health subcultures of the public? Since empirical evidence suggests that social policies do not have a great impact on 'health behaviour', something must be wrong with these interrelationships.

The relationship between health subcultures and social policy sectors

In exploring the relationship between social policy makers and subcultures it is clear that we need to know more about the relationship between the micro level of 'social health' and the macro level of 'societal health'. We need to know how social policies relate to the gap between these two.

In an empirical study on health, the family, and utilization of formal and informal services in my region (560 families in Emilia-Romagna, Italy), health subcultures were related to use of the health services provided. The health subcultures were derived empirically by factor analysis. They are characterized as follows. The organic subculture refers to beliefs and practices which consider health to be linked to such factors as a subjective perception of well-being, looking good, eating healthy food, and sleeping regularly. The medicalized subculture sees health as intrinsically related to frequent visits to the doctor, testing, screening, and taking medicines. The relational subculture understands health as being at peace with the world, avoiding stress, having good interpersonal relations, being socially integrated, enjoying a pollution-free environment, and so on. The health services considered come from different sources: informal networks, market, and the state.

The analyses clearly show that the organic subculture is strongly correlated with the existence and daily use of effective social support networks. The medicalized subculture is especially linked to the use of private or 'for profit' services. The relational subculture is prevalent among those social groups which rely heavily upon public services.

The social processes can be elucidated further. It is apparent that people do not have sufficient resources and supports to practice healthy behaviour under pressure from conditioning factors such as mass media and the regulated market. These pressures need to be counteracted by supporting agencies such as informal networks and not-for-profit associations which can reduce imbalances. Social policies must therefore consist of measures increasing the power of individuals enabling resistance to those forces which aim to make individuals, groups, and communities more and more dependent upon alienating factors. Alienating factors may come from the submerged economy such as those forcing people to work in bad and dangerous conditions. There are those from the regulated market, such as the sales promotion of drugs; from the mass media, advertising of alcohol and cigarettes for example; and from unresponsive institutional services, inhumane hospitals, children in institutions.

The role of formal services in health behaviour

The relationship between the utilization of health and social services to health behaviour will now be considered. At the University of Bologna surveys on 'health education and the use of health services' are currently being carried out.

Health behaviour is conceived as the product of a complex interchange of factors linked to the individual's life style on the one hand and to the utilization of formal services on the other. The links between these can be direct or mediated by the subject.

From the social policy perspective we must know more about the impact of the welfare state on individual life style and the utilization of social and health services if we want to explain health behaviour. Within this framework, an important theme is the links and interrelationships between formal and informal solutions in meeting health needs. Much evidence exists that these different ways of coping with health problems are quantitatively comparable, and that people prefer combinatory solutions rather than alternative resorts.

Statistical data from the research previously mentioned gives an idea of the importance of the use of formal services. Table 20.1 clearly shows that the utilization of formal services, medicalized behaviours, the utilization of the family doctor, and health self-control, are related to gender and age. Table 20.2 shows how the same variables vary along with social stratification, level of education, and the family life cycle. These correlations must be

Table 20.1 Some statistical data from a survey in Emilia-Romagna, stratified random sample of 560 families (1985)*

Index of (range 0–4)	Gender		Mean
	Males	Females	
Utilization of formal services	1.26	1.71	1.48
Medicalized behaviour	0.21	0.16	0.19
Family doctor utilization	1.43	1.31	1.37
Health self- control	0.85	1.43	1.13

	Age						Mean
	18–24	24–34	35–44	45–54	55–64	65+	
Utilization of formal services	1.57	1.44	1.11	1.76	1.38	1.88	1.48
Medicalized behaviour	0.06	0.17	0.19	0.33	0.22	0.77	0.19
Family doctor utilization	1.01	1.29	1.61	1.82	1.38	2.33	1.37
Health self-control	0.98	1.28	0.98	1.35	1.02	1.22	1.13

* Details of the scaling and scoring systems are available from the author.

understood in connection with the existence and functioning of informal networks. This illustrates the value of gathering data and interpreting it in relation to the family as a unit of reference for health behaviour. To this end a national survey of about 30 000 households in Italy is planned with the aim of relating health behaviour to the whole family situation and quality of life.

The old dilemma of universalistic *vs.* selective measures

The link between research and action and the relationship between universalisitic intervention, as opposed to selective measures, are illustrated in Fig. 20.1.

It is evident that we need more research on the whole population as well as on targeted groups from the intervention or social policy perspective. Legal procedures can reduce risk factors via universalistic measures but particular groups still remain with their unanswered troubles. There must be corresponding positively discriminating selective measures which can help vested interests and disadvantaged groups to emerge and set up their own security system in order to promote health.

Table 20.2 Other statistical data on health behaviour and the utilization of health services (above-mentioned research)

	Index of (range 0–4)			
	Utilization of formal services	Medicalized behaviour	Family doctor utilization	Health self-control
Social class				
Upper	1.37	0.06	0.80	1.37
Middle	1.46	0.14	1.20	1.14
Low	1.60	0.54	1.94	1.33
Marginals	1.66	0.05	1.16	1.16
Mean	1.48	0.19	1.37	1.13
Education				
High	1.39	0.02	0.78	1.43
Middle	1.55	0.08	1.07	1.09
Low	1.12	0.87	2.62	0.62
Mean	1.48	0.79	1.37	1.13
Family life cycle				
Single or couple with no children	1.19	0.46	1.51	1.34
Couple with children aged up to 5	1.36	—	0.84	0.94
Couple with children 6–14	1.34	0.10	1.22	1.16
Couple with adult children	1.57	0.15	1.39	1.10
Old couple alone	1.55	0.22	1.33	0.88
Old person alone	1.51	0.50	2.00	0.50
Mean	1.48	1.19	1.37	1.13

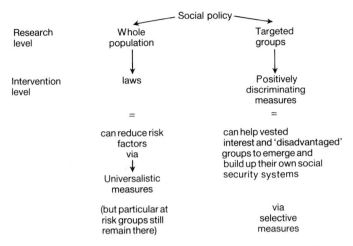

Fig. 20.1 The structures of social policy as a differentiated process oriented towards 'health for all'.

Old and new queries

The assessment, promotion, and support of health behaviour in the perspective of social policy depends upon several factors:

1. A renewal of public participation in health services, both informal and formal, but especially at the local level.
2. A renewal of prevention, especially primary prevention, through an involvement of life-world agencies such as teachers in schools, workers in factories, parents in the family.
3. An increased reponsibility of the consumers or 'prosumers'.
4. Proper utilization of the new telematic media.
5. A new responsibility for health professionals.

There are many queries relating to these. It is not clear how participation can be promoted in each of the different sectors. Presumably the means of promotion will differ in each sector, although the differences remain to be expounded. A reappraisal of action research in this field is perhaps desirable. In renewing prevention the peculiarities of potential agencies need to be explored. Their relative abilities and responsibilities need more accurate description in order that they be effectively mobilized. An analysis of legislation on health education and the involvement of such agencies is required. In attempts to increase the responsibility of the consumers we must consider barriers to approaching bureaucracies and examine the possibility of legitimizing the social support networks as an autonomous sector of the health services and thus as a field for action beyond the state and the market. Proper utilization of new telematic media must consider fostering a more efficient and effective use of formal and informal services and the possibility for enhancing social networks of particular groups. There has already been a 'teleaid' project aimed at the elderly in Italy. The health professionals need to consider equity and reciprocity, and to take steps towards symmetry in the relationship between professionals and clients. A new differentiation of the medical role brought about by positive sanctionings of new health-oriented profiles in medical careers would perhaps be a step towards this end.

The general conclusions of this chapter are as follows. The concept of healthy life style must be examined more closely. More specifically we must consider whether it is possible to think of social policies oriented towards healthy life styles as normal life styles. If it is possible to agree on a new concept of 'normality' as an adequate relation to the social environment and to the generalized alter, what are the implications of this? For instance, is it possible to think of social policies which are able to reward health behaviour instead of compensating for illness a posteriori? Above all we need means of treating the community as a system for formal and informal relations as such, and we must assess urgently how the so-called health system does in fact work to produce full health by avoiding negative, unattended, or perverse outcomes.

References

Donati, P. (ed.) (1983a). *La sociologia sanitaria. Dalla sociologia della medicina alla sociologia della salute*. F. Angeli, Milano.

Donati, P. (ed.) (1983b). La nuova sociologia della salute. In *Introduzione alla sociologia relazionale*. F. Angeli, Milano.

Donati, P. (1984). *Risposte alla crisi dello Stato sociale*. F. Angeli, Milano.

Donati, P. (ed.) (1985). *Le frontiere della politica sociale. Redistribuzione e nuova cittadinanza*. F. Angeli, Milano.

21

Directions for research in health behaviour related to health promotion: an overview

DAVID V. MCQUEEN

Introduction

The field of health-behaviour research is multidisciplinary and extensive, as is witnessed by the range of interests represented in this book. Thus, it should be remarked at the outset of this chapter, that it is not possible to consider priorities and strategies for health-behaviour research in a manner which would encompass this vast field. Instead, the focus of this chapter is about directions for health-behaviour research *as applied to health promotion*. A second caveat is that any discussion of research priorities and needs will reflect the background and interests of the author. In the tradition of *reflexive sociology* , one should state at the outset one's prejudices about the conduct of research. In my own case, I believe that research in health-related behaviour should be eclectic, combining both qualitative and quantitative approaches, with a multidisciplinary perspective.* Further, I believe there is little room for individual researchers who believe they have a special 'insight' on how to ascertain the truth about health and about behaviour related to health. It is fundamental to recognize that the current state of research is largely atheoretical, and rather primitive methodologically. Therefore, some of the most pressing issues involve basic research questions of theory and method. This chapter offers one perspective on these issues.

It could be argued that health-behaviour research has advanced con-siderably since the middle of the century. I would assert that the question of 'progress' in health-behaviour research remains open. Much of what appears as advancement may be mere changes in research directions or 'fashions'. For example, every decade brings new conceptual emphases. The emphasis of the present decade has shifted from a focus on individual behaviour to a concern with the context of behaviour. This emphasis is best illustrated by current interest in research on 'life style' and 'contextualism'.

---

* This chapter is mainly concerned with quantitative research in health. The issues, problems, and methods of qualitative research are not discussed. Multidisciplinary is meant to include the disciplines of both the social and natural sciences.

Traditionally, most research in health behaviour has been dominated by ideologies and methods which developed in public health and the social sciences. To a great extent these endeavours have followed 'classical' research designs propounded by the natural sciences. The result has been a marked dependency on survey techniques, quasi-experimental designs, case-control studies, and other 'static' designs. It is often characterized by brief periods of intensive 'data-collection', followed by long periods of analysis which ultimately result in a voluminous report (e.g. the 'grey' literature of government documents). These research 'results' often constitute an extensive, elaborate, and usually accurate picture of health attitudes, opinions, and behaviours at the point of data collection. But they are simply 'snapshots' of a group, culture, or nation at one moment in time. It is not 'dynamic' and it is therefore not surprising that, despite the considerable amount of extant 'health-behaviour research', we still know relatively little about the process and dynamics of health-related behavioural change.

Clearly, research in health behaviour which follows 'classical' approaches should not be suspended. Much has been learned and that knowledge should be applied. There is now a need to turn to more dynamic, less 'traditional' research designs which can detect changing patterns of health-related behaviours. Fortunately there is a growing body of literature, both theoretical and methodological, which is concerned with the problem of change over time. On balance, the theoretical arguments are not well developed, but the methodological techniques for exploring continuous data are becoming available. It is a challenge for the health research community to adapt to them as it did to the traditional methods.

Theories, definitions, and behaviour

Research in health-related behaviour has suffered particularly from a lack of theory and an inability to agree upon definitions of key concepts, including the meaning of health behaviour itself. Theory is most crucial: it serves as a guide and prevents health researchers from engaging in 'raw empiricism'. No doubt every survey researcher has designed over-long questionnaires solely on the rationale to 'get it while you're there'. Rarely does one collect data because it is necessary to accept or reject an hypothesis which derives from a theory. The lack of theory often results in an enormous data-set which, when extensively manipulated or massaged, yields many statistically significant correlations, but proves very little.

A theory of behaviour might consider three elements: (a) the nature of human development; (b) the role of the environment (social and physical); and (c) the interaction of development and environment. Unfortunately most theoretical work has focused narrowly on either the first or the second component. Development of behaviour as a product of the individual's genetic code has been largely a domain of natural scientists. Animal studies, notably by ethologists, have revealed many of the elaborate behaviour patterns of higher order animals; attempts to view human behaviour in the same light have led to considerable understanding of development. This literature on development is particularly rich in understanding the early years of human growth. The behavioural repertoire of adults is less understood and exacerbated significantly by complex social factors stemming from the social environment. A theory of behaviour considering these three elements poses several questions for researchers concerned with behaviour: (*a*) what are the patterns of health-related behaviours during an individual's life span; (*b*) to what extent are these patterns linked to a particular social environment; and (*c*) to what extent do particular groups, cohorts, and nations differ in behaviours. The answers to these questions present issues of practical application as well as ethical issues because adequate answers could form the bases for the appropriate targeting of health-promotion efforts.

Recently, Featherman and Lerner (1985) proposed a theory with implications for 'life span' research which attempts to consider the three elements above. Although the general notion of life span research is not particularly new (for example Erikson 1959, 1963; Havighurst 1952; Neugarten 1968), Featherman and Lerner (p. 660) argue for a 'conceptualization of development of a bi-directional, person population process'. Their derived conceptual scheme of development as a population process is quite complex but includes three 'ecological levels', the institutional, the behavioural, and the biogenetic. These are viewed both from their static and processual characteristics. They contend that '... the place of a person or group in the social structure of a given society ... condition the likelihood that development in some behavioural dimension will occur, what pattern it will take, and when it will begin and end in a personal biography or history of a collectivity' (p. 664). Although their theoretical development provides stimulating reading, their methodological suggestions for research remain problematic.

A major problem with a development or 'life span' approach is that it tends to overemphasize the role of the individual as a biological entity at the expense of how the individual relates to the social environment. In Edinburgh we are pursuing a theory, drawing upon many studies in psychophysiology and cognitive psychology, which argues that activities which are habitually performed become 'routine', such that higher level cognitive processing is, for most of the time, unnecessary. Such activities are therefore carried out with a minimum of awareness, coming to the forefront of consciousness only occasionally. The behaviour involved in smoking, drinking, the buying, eating and preparation of food, physical exercise, is built into the flow of daily life in a largely routine way, with these behaviours resulting in predictable and relatively stable individual patterns. This relegation of habits to lower levels of consciousness may be seen as part of a general adaptation process which allows the person to deal with a potentially huge number of internal and external events, so that decision-making processes are free to deal with the more novel and salient features of daily life.

Another aspect of this adaptation process is 'selective perception' whereby only those stimuli and issues which have relevance for the individual in his/her immediate surrounding or primary group are attended to and non-salient information does not reach awareness. In other words, each individual carries some implicit 'world of meaning' which has a profound effect on what kinds of information gets through. Further elements in adaptation are the ability of the individual to deal with environmental contingencies, the coping strategies available, and the extent to which these strategies are being taxed. It may be asserted that there are many worlds of meaning possessed by an individual, not the least of which is that world of meaning which contains beliefs, values, and attitudes regarding health and illness. Furthermore there may well be coping strategies particular to these health beliefs.

There is evidence that spontaneous behavioural change occurs when some formerly routine activity is brought into awareness for a prolonged period of time—i.e. it becomes salient or problematic. This often occurs in conjunction with a change in the context in which the behaviour in question is being carried out. For example, a smoker going to live with a non-smoker. The actions associated with a former 'habit' are now subject to 'cognitive appraisal'. It is argued that this new awareness leads to a change in selective perception and, thus, that which was formerly 'unseen' now impinges on consciousness as the event or information changes its meaning (Hunt and Martin 1988).

These two examples of theory in behavioural research illustrate how theories stemming from various disciplines might be brought to bear on the specific problem of research in health behaviour related to health promotion. Whether or not a distinctive theory which applies uniquely to health-related behaviour is possible, remains an open question. Obviously, one major need in health-behaviour research is attention to this question.

Definitional problems abound in the literature on health behaviour. For *heuristic* purposes health behaviours may be divided into three 'types'. Roughly categorized, *health-enhancing behaviours* correspond chiefly to behaviours concerned with health promotion, i.e. those behaviours which are conscious attempts to improve one's level of overall health. The use of the term health enhancement has been widely adopted by WHO and many researchers concerned with the area of health promotion. A full explication of this terminology and its historical development is found in several chapters of a recent handbook on health enhancement (Matarazzo *et al.* 1984). *Health-maintaining behaviours* are generally conceived as behaviours related to prevention. Many such behaviours are often independent of the formal medical care system (e.g. self-care, the routine use of vitamins, etc.), but others (e.g. immunization, screening) do require limited interaction with organized medical care. Finally, *health-damaging behaviours* include those which could be considered as negative health behaviours. Found among these behaviours are the traditional behavioural 'risk factors' for disease (e.g. smoking, drinking, drug abuse, etc.).

What health behaviours need to be considered in health-promotion research? One could simply list a series of behaviours; numerous listings of health-related behaviours have been published, but in reality the challenge isn't simply to itemize behaviours. The research need is to measure important health-related behaviours reliably and validly and to understand the social contexts in which they take place. Each category of behaviour requires consideration with respect to currently used measurement methods and the extent to which improvement is required on widely used items attempting to measure health behaviour. To illustrate this problem, consider the 'appetitive' area of behaviour, with drinking and smoking behaviour as examples of the health-related behaviours. Although difficulties remain with the measurement of alcohol intake of individuals, it can be argued that the sources of error are understood and that valid estimates are possible (Celentano and McQueen 1978). In a similar vein, smoking behaviour and its measurement has been highly refined. Taken separately, the measurements of alcohol and tobacco use are quite standard. None the less, they are of limited use to us. The concern of health-behaviour research is the development of a composite, i.e. integrated measure of substance use and abuse which takes into account the processual interactions among the substances under study. The aim should be to incorporate the *context* of use into a measure and take into account the interactions among the behaviours. Ultimately the goal is to understand how these behavioural components change relative to one another over time. Thus, when interactions, context, and change are taken into account, questionnaire items which had previously been accepted by researchers as valid and reliable in assessing one behaviour at one point in time, will be in need of significant modification.

Life style has been a buzzword in health-related research for several years.* This all-embracing concept appears to be largely defined by a

---

* The concept of 'life-style' is at present seemingly vague. None the less, a theory of life style should be developed. At present the behavioural interpretation of life style remains very controversial, thus any life-style theory will in turn be considered with much scepticism. At the centre of this controversy, although never expressed in these terms, is the classic question of universals, the familiar realism–nominalism continuum. Is life style simply a convenient word on which to hang specific behavioural examples, or is it a concept which provides a coherent picture of human behavioural reality? Perhaps there is a life-style 'state'. In the traditional social science paradigm, there is specification of what exactly the behaviour of an actor is. Life-style theory substitutes this problematic assumption by a formulation which specifies how the life-style state changes in abstract space. What, however, is actually observed is not the life style state, but the actor behaving in real space. Life-style theory connects the life-style state and the status of the

constellation of behaviours conducive to good health (Anderson 1984; Dean 1984; Robertson 1984). Part of the groundwork for this notion stems from a quarter century of extensive research in the NIH-funded Human Population Laboratory at Berkeley, California. Often referred to as the 'Alameda' study, this multidisciplinary work examined people's social networks, sleeping and eating patterns, smoking behaviours, alcohol use, and community participation. The results of this work, recently summarized in Berkman and Breslow (1983), indicated that there is a strong causal relationship between ways of living and both morbidity and mortality. Partly because of these findings, the notion of 'life style' has become almost as accepted among many health researchers as the 'traditional' risk factors such as socio-economic status, age, sex, etc. Despite the apparent success of this approach many researchers have questioned components of the concept (e.g. Wiley and Comacho 1980; Taylor and Ford 1981), and many have pointed out the vagueness of the notion. Attempts to clarify the notion abound, for example Milio (1981) defines life styles as 'patterns of (behavioural) choices made from the alternatives that are available to people according to their socio-economic circumstances and to the ease with which they are able to choose certain ones over others.' Clearly such definitions remain problematic for researchers who must try and operationalize such a notion into a unit of analysis. None the less, implicit in the notion are many of the issues which link behaviour to health and it would be difficult for future research in health and behaviour to dismiss easily the idea that 'life style' bears a causal relationship to health status.

The life-style concept implies an important role for socio-environmental factors. However, the role of social factors in *specific behaviours* related to a 'healthy life style' remains unclear. One reason lies in the difficult problem of conceptualizing and measuring such a macro construct as the 'social environment'. No single study can hope to provide information on all components of the social environment which are assumed to relate to health behaviours.

---

actor in real space in terms of probability. What happens when we measure human behaviour? Just after the measurement we have considerable information, and more than provided by the notion of life-style state. The life-style state only told us that the actor had a certain probability of being in a certain status. In taking a measurement we destroy the current life-style state and replace it with a new one which has all the probability at the point where we measured the actor. The sudden, discontinuous change of the life-style state following measurement is the 'collapse of the life-style state'. Thus there are two ways in which the life-style state can change in time. Most of the time it changes smoothly and deterministically. However, just after a measurement has taken place, it must jump into a new life-style state to agree with the results of the measurement. The life-style concept is very different from the concept that the social science paradigm was meant to describe. In particular, life-style systems have a certain 'wholeness (plenum)'. Because of this irreducibility we cannot give a complete description of a system by breaking it down into its parts, as one does in traditional social science. Once two actors interact, they become part of one social system, and we cannot describe this system completely merely by giving a complete description of the two actors individually.

These components include: socio-economic status; demographic factors; social network; and the less tangible variables such as social support, social integration, psychosocial stress, and other variables which incorporate social relationships. Obviously these components are themselves multidimensional and interactive. Consider the example of socio-economic status, which in western sociology is generally conceived as related to where one lives, one's occupation, one's educational background, and one's disposable income. Further the immediate environment (housing quality, family structure, access to shops, social support, etc.) is highly influenced by one's socio-economic status. Fortunately, there is a wealth of relevant research literature which has contended with many of these social environmental factors (e.g. for Britain see Blaxter 1981; Blaxter and Paterson 1982; Brown and Harris 1978; Carter and Peel 1976; Halsey 1981; Rappaport *et al*. 1982; Rutter and Madja 1976; Townsend and Davidson 1982). [For a recent review of this area see Macintyre 1986.] Despite this extensive literature, major questions remain unanswered with respect to health behaviours and social factors, even within western sociological traditions. From the standpoint of health-promotion research there is a need to understand how the three types of behaviours (health enhancing, damaging, and maintaining) relate to and are causally related to these well known social factors.

Methodological issues

Historically, cross-sectional surveys have dominated research in the field of behavioural research. However, such an approach will not easily detect change and a longitudinal and/or panel design is usually deemed necessary. There are, however, new data collection and analysis possibilities which may be applicable to the study of behavioural change—for example, through the continuous collection of data.

In order to study short-term changes in behaviour and to account for periodic differences, one strategy might be to collect data in short 'bursts' and, in the ideal case, 52 weeks during the year. The brief periods in between 'bursts' would be utilized to review the data received to date and allow for strategic adjustments in questions asked. Thus, the research would be responsive to current changes in behaviours. This 'burst' method of data collection requires a data management approach. Such an approach is conceptually more like taking an 'inventory', in this case an inventory of behaviours. Fortunately, the current state of computer technology makes such an approach feasible, especially with the possibility of daily on-line entry of data.

Once individuals became part of such a study they would become a resource for information on both long-term and short-term behavioural patterns. Thus, once interviewed, they would expect to be re-interviewed, by telephone, postal, or face-to-face methods, at least yearly and some more often. Further, quarterly subsamples on special topics, with brief interviews, would be possible in order to assess changes resulting from some particular event, e.g. a government report on smoking or a national health education campaign.

Collecting data on a continuous basis presents many research issues which need to be faced. From a technical point of view, the main issues revolve around sampling, data management, methods of data collection, and units of analysis. The sampling issues are beyond the scope of this presentation and involve some very basic questions about the nature of research in the behavioural sciences. It is clear that new methods of sampling need to be explored and should themselves be a subject of study. This is not wholly disconnected from the problem of data collection. If, for example, the telephone is used to collect data and a random digit dialling technique (such as the Waksberg method) is used, then sampling and information gathering become coterminous. The work of Hogelin (q.v.) represents work in health-behaviour research applied to health promotion which has dealt with these issues. In Edinburgh, the Women's Health Shop Study used combined telephone sampling and data collection techniques. The technical problems associated with such research should be given priority in health-behaviour research because they are fundamental to the development of a 'dynamic' model of behavioural change.

Methodological aims of data collection include representativeness, validity and reliability of measurement and, in analysis, causality. In seeking to achieve this, new problems have arisen. To illustrate, in data collection more emphasis has had to be placed on the 'mode' of collection. Questions of cost-effectiveness, interviewer bias, and interviewer safety have led to the employment of postal and telephone methods. Where telephone ownership is limited, mixed 'mode' methods have been developed. In general, concern has shifted to the problem of total survey error (Lessler 1979) arising from sampling variability, non-sampling variability, response effects, and non-participation effects. The latter is a special problem, as both American and European studies have noted an increase in non-response rates (Dalenius 1977, 1979). Many non-statistical techniques such as call-backs, encouragement, substitution, and promise of confidentiality, have been used with varying success; in addition, statistical techniques such as weighting for missing data (Tupek and Richardson 1978) and imputation techniques (Rubin 1978, 1979) are being developed to account for data collection variability (Tanur 1983).

Multiple units of analysis

One of the most pressing problems is that data in research on behaviours are often presented or collected at two or more levels of observation. Historically, many social science researchers have tended to ignore this problem and lumped all the units of analysis together. Thus data on individuals are simply aggregated into data on groups. Often the 'levels' of the units are not conceptualized as different and such conceptual entities as 'individuals', 'households', and 'neighbourhoods' are simply linked together as if they were the same kinds of units from a measurement standpoint. Perhaps this is because the distinctions are not as conceptually distinctive as units of analysis in the natural sciences (e.g. in biology—the molecular, cellular, tissue, organ levels). In addition, the statistical underpinnings of multilevel analysis (Lindley and Smith 1972) are beyond the scope of most social scientists. Recently, Mason Wong, and Entwistle (1983) have made efforts to bring these analytical considerations to the attention of sociologists. The underlying strategy is 'the notion of a regression in which the dependent variable consists of regression coefficients from other regressions . . .' (p. 73). The need for such techniques in the study of behaviour related to health is self-evident, owing to the fact that our data is often a mixture of different levels of data. But such strategies, if they are to be employed, require a multi-disciplinary and perhaps a multi-centre approach (i.e. involving research centres with different kinds of expertise, and experience with different levels of variables). The future developments of such techniques may well be crucial to the very 'essence' of health promotion. Conceptually, health promotion has made a strong case that it is not concerned with 'just' individual behaviour, but also with social processes which are larger than the individual. None the less, data are usually collected only on individual behaviours and self reports of perceptions of social processes. These different conceptual 'levels' are then treated as if they are one.

Methodological issues cannot be separated from the problems which are implied in the concept of 'contextualism'. This is apparent in the role of contextual factors which relate to the capacity of an individual to muster social mechanisms of defence to alter a pathological process (for an extensive discussion of this idea see McQueen and Celentano 1982). Here one is dealing with several variable clusters which have been, and continue to be, major subjects of research related to behaviour and health, namely: social networks, social support, and social processes. Because the current state of research on these subjects probably includes the majority of studies in health and social behaviour it would be foolish to attempt a review of it here (compare Dean 1986; Kaplan *et al.* 1983; House *et al.* 1982). Suffice it to say that these concepts are seen as vital to understanding health behaviour. None the less, the vast majority of this research has been concerned with chronic disease, principally coronary heart disease and mental health (notably depression), and relatively little has been devoted to health-related behaviour and its change.

A recent paper by Westman, Eden, and Shirom (1985) on smoking cessation is illustrative of a study incorporating 'contextual effects'. Working at Tel Aviv University with the Cardiac Evaluation and Rehabilitation Institute in Tel Hashomer (the multi-centre, multi-discipline approach), they studied several hundred disease-free male smokers. They used multiple regression techniques of analysis and argued the main-effect hypothesis that stress is positively related to smoking intensity and negatively to cessation. Variables of interest measured in the study included: job stress (role conflict, quantitative role overload, responsibility for persons, hours of work, social pressure, intrinsic impoverishment, lack of participation, lack of influence, harsh working conditions); peer support; smoking cessation; and smoking intensity (number of cigarettes smoked per day). They argue, with respect to social support [just one factor]:

If the supportive others are nonsmokers and nonsmoking norms prevail among one's peers at work, then the conventional social support buffer hypothesis is tenable. Bolstered by such supporters, a smoker can be expected to withstand greater job stress without resorting to intensification of smoking as an aid to coping and efforts to cease smoking would have greater likelihood of succeeding. However, when smoking peers are a significant source of support, their support can be expected to throttle his smoking when under high or low job stress, perhaps via a social facilitation process . . . Thus, social support for the smoker under stress may be a double-edged sword, and should be studied as such in the future (p. 643).

This type of research shows the complexity of studying some notion such as smoking cessation within the context of a real-life situation, namely the workplace. It also illustrates the need for relatively confined 'micro studies' which elaborate a complex relationship within a sharply defined setting. It does attempt to explain individual behaviour in terms of some different level social processes. The fruits of such research for future health-promotion intervention strategies lie in a better articulation of the interplay among levels of analysis.

The social factor principle* is premised on a notion of causality. Implied in

* The conceptualization of the 'social factors principle' is very complex and would include a large literature and tradition in research on health-related behaviour. To begin with there is nothing set in stone with respect to this terminology. There are many alternative phrases which could convey a similar meaning to the one chosen. For example, for the word 'social' one could substitute 'socio-cultural', 'psychosocial', 'socio-economic', and so forth. For the word 'factor' one could substitute 'processes', 'aspects', 'contexts'. In stressing *social* factors it is also recognized that man is a biological being. Whereas biology cheifly concerns itself with the interface of man with his physical environment, the social sciences primarily consider the interactions of the social being with the external society. Several basic tenets with respect to the

the approach is the idea that the 'factor' causes a process to occur. Current methodological strategies in social epidemiology and behavioural science emphasize causal modeling. ['Causal modeling is a technique for selecting those variables that are potential determinants of the effects and then attempting to isolate the separate contributions to the effects made by each predictor variable' (Asher 1976).] The statistical techniques for the required multivariate designs have been extensively developed in the past 15–20 years. Pioneering work in this field has been conducted by Blalock (1964, 1968), Goodman (1973), and Land (1969). The coterminous development of computer hardware and software has facilitated the use of these techniques by social scientists, now seen in the common use of multiple regression, path analysis, log-linear analysis and *Lisrel* by social scientists (Joreskog and Sorbom 1982; Alwin and Hauser 1975; Kessler and Greenberg 1981; Henry 1982). Only recently, however, has attention been paid to such applications with discrete data (Feinberg 1980; Goodman 1979; Winship and Mare 1983). The state of the art indicates the feasibility of such causal modeling for data on behaviour related to health. The question remains of how this wealth of methodological technique can be integrated into health-behaviour research linked to health promotion.

Conclusions

A major challenge for health-behaviour research in its application to health promotion is how to link theory, methods, and empirical research in health behaviour to health promotion. Two general questions should be considered:

1. 'Do we develop theory and methods to conduct research into behavioural change in order to understand how health promotion might be more effectively applied or targeted?'
2. 'Do we study health-related behaviour and its change over time in order to detect the impact of health promotion to bring about these changes?'

The former is *basic* research which informs policy for health promotion; the latter is *evaluation* of health promotion. Although in practice these can only be artificially divorced from each other, from a research perspective the two questions generate quite distinctive research hypotheses.* For example,

---

social being and its interface with the external society are: (*a*) we are located within society and this determines and defines most of what we do; (*b*) society is an objective external factor which cannot be denied and is coercive in its control over us; (*c*) society contains institutions which pattern our actions and modes of behaviour; (*d*) most importantly, even biological reality takes on meaning only when it is socially interpreted by individuals.

 * This distinction is reminiscent of the now long-playing argument over sociology *in* medicine versus sociology *of* medicine. Such philosophical exegeses, while not a concern of this chapter, are necessary if research related to health promotion is to come of age.

basic research in behaviour related to health promotion will be concerned with such hypotheses as:

- Individuals will have consistent patterns of health behaviour in terms of the enhancing/maintaining/risk typology.
- Social environmental factors (e.g. housing, employment status) will be associated with health behaviour.
- Cohort effects in health behaviours will be discernable.
- Type and 'level' of health behaviours will differ significantly with an individual's stage in the lifespan.
- There will be marked differences in health behaviours in relation to geographical location of subjects.
- The concept of 'life style' is a unique variable which relates to behavioural change and health-related patterns.

Evaluation of health promotion will generate quite different research hypotheses, such as:

- Specific health-promotion programmes will be associated with changes in specific types of health behaviour.
- Socio-economic status will predict statistically significant differences in types of health behaviours in response to health promotion.
- The social 'context' of behaviour can be manipulated by health-promotion strategies and lead to health-enhancing behaviours.

It is hoped that the combined chapters of this book will lead to numerous research questions of value and that they will serve as a guide for health-behaviour related to health promotion.

References

Alwin, D. F. and Hauser, R. M. (1975). The decomposition of effects in path analysis. *American Sociological Review* **40**, 37–47.

Anderson, R. (1984). Health promotion: an overview. *European Monographs in Health Education Research* **6**, 1–76.

Asher, H. B. (1976). *Causal Modeling*. Sage Publications, London.

Berkman, L. F. and Breslow, L. (1983). *Health and ways of living: the Alameda County Study*. Oxford University Press, New York.

Blalock, H. M. Jr (1964). *Causal inferences in non-experimental research*. University of North Carolina Press, Chapel Hill.

Blalock, H. M. Jr (1968). Theory building and causal inferences. In *Methodology in Social Research* (eds H. M. Blalock and A. B. Blalock). McGraw-Hill, New York.

Blaxter, M. (1981). *The health of children*. Heinemann Educational, London.

Blaxter, M. and Paterson, E. (1982). *Mothers and daughters: a three generational study of health attitudes and behaviour*. Heinemann Educational, London.

Bradburn, N. M. and Sudman, S. (1981). *Improving interview method and question-naire design*. Jossey-Bass Publishers, London.

Brown, G. W. and Harris, T. O. (1978). *Social origins of depression*. Tavistock Publications, London.

Cannell, C. F., Miller, P. V., and Oksenberg, L. (1981). Research on interviewing techniques. In *Sociological methodology* (ed. S. Leinhardt), pp. 389–437. Jossey-Bass Publishers, San Francisco.

Carter, C. O. and Peel, J. (1976). *Equalities and inequalities in health*. Academic Press, London.

Celentano, D. D. and McQueen, D. V. (1976). Comparison of alcoholism prevalence rates obtained by survey and indirect estimators. *Journal of Studies on Alcohol* **39**, 420–34.

Celentano, D. D. and McQueen, D. V. (1978). Reliability and validity of alcoholism prevalence estimators. *Journal of Studies on Alcohol* **39**, 000–000.

Dalenius, T. (1977). Bibliography on non-sampling errors in surveys. *International Statistical Institute Review* **45**, 71–90, 181–97, 303–17.

Dalenius, T. (1979). Informed consent or R.S.V.P. Panel on Incomplete Data of the Committee on National Statistics/National Research Council. In *Symposium on Incomplete Data: Preliminary Proceedings*, pp. 94–134. Washington, D.C.: U.S. Dept. of Health, Education and Welfare, Social Security Administration, Office of Policy, Office of Research and Statistics.

Dean, K. (1984). Influence of health beliefs on lifestyles: what do we know? *European Monographs in Health Education Research* **6**, 127–49.

Dean, K. (1986). Social support and health: pathways of influence. *Health Promotion* **1**, 133–50.

Erikson, E. H. (1959). Identity and the life cycle (selected papers). In *Psychological Issues* (ed. G. S. Klein). International Universities Press, New York/

Featherman, D. L. and Lerner, R. M. (1985). Ontogenesis and sociogenesis: prob-lematics for theory and research about development and socialization across the lifespan. *American Sociological Review* **50**, 659–76.

Feinberg, S. E. (1980). *The analysis of cross-classified categorical data* 2nd edn. MIT Press, Cambridge.

Goodman, L. A. (1973). Causal analysis of data from panel studies and other kinds of surveys. *American Journal of Sociology* **78**, 1135–91.

Goodman, L. A. (1979). A brief guide to the causal analysis of data from surveys. *American Journal of Sociology* **84**, 1078–95.

Halsey, A. H. (1981). *Changes in British Society*, Tavistock, London.

Havighurst, R. (1952). *Developmental tasks and education* Longmans Green, New York.

Henry, J. P. (1982). The relation of social to biological processes in disease. *Social Science and Medicine* **16**–80.

House, J. S. *et al.* (1982). The association of social relationships and activities with mortality: prospective evidence from the Tecumseh community health study. *American Journal of Epidemiology* **116**, 123–40.

Hunt, S. M. and Martin, C. J. (1988). Health-related behavioural change: A pre-liminary test of a new model. *Psychology and Health* (In Press).

Joreskog, K. and Sorbom, D. (1982). *LISREL V: Analysis of linear structural relationships by the method of maximum likelihood*. International Educational Services, Chicago.

Kaplan, B. H. *et al*. (1983). The epidemiologic evidence for a relationship between social support and health. *American Journal of Epidemiology* **117**, 521–37.

Kessler, R. C. and Greenberg, D. F. (1981). *Linear panel analysis: models of quantitative change*. Academic Press, New York.

Kickbusch, I. (1986). Life-styles and health. *Social Science and Medicine* **22**, 117–24.

Land, K. C. (1969). Principles of path analysis. In *Sociological methodology* (ed. E. Borgatta), pp. 3–37. Jossey-Bass Publishers, San Francisco.

Lessler, J. R. (1979). An expanded survey error model. Panel on Incomplete Data of the Committee on National Statistics/National Research Council, In *Symposium on Incomplete Data: Preliminary Proceedings*. Washington, D.C.: U.S. Department of Health, Education and Welfare, Social Security Administrative Office of Policy, Office of Research and Statistics.

Lindley, D. V. and Smith, A. F. M. (1972). Bayes estimates for the linear model. (with discussion). *Journal of the Royal Statistical Society*, Series B **34**, 1–41.

Macintyre, S. (1986). The patterning of health by social position in contemporary Britain; directions for sociological research. *Social Science and Medicine* **23**, (4), pp. 393–415.

McQueen, D. V. and Celentano, D. D. (1982). Social factors in the etiology of multiple outcomes. *Social Science and Medicine* **16**, 397–418.

McQueen, D. V. and Siegrist, J. (1982). Social factors in the etiology of chronic disease: and overview. *Social Science and Medicine* **16**, 353–67.

Mason, W. M., Wong, G. Y., and Entwistle, B. (1983). Contextual analysis through the multilevel linear model. In *Sociological Methodology* (ed. S. Leinhardt). Jossey-Bass Publishers, London.

Matarazzo, J. D. *et al*. (eds) (1984). *Behavioural health: a handbook of health enhancement and disease prevention*. John Wiley and Sons, New York.

Milio, N. (1981). *Promoting Health Through Public Policy*. F. A. Davis, Philadelphia.

Miller, P. V. and Cannell, C. F. (1982). A study of experimental techniques for telephone interviewing. *Public Opinion Quarterly* **46**, 250–69.

Neugarten, B. L. (1968). The awareness of middle age. In *Middle age and aging* (Chapter 10). University of Chicago Press.

Pearlin, L. I. (1982). Discontinuities in the study of ageing. In *Ageing and life course transitions: an interdisciplinary perspective* (Chapter 3). Tavistock, London.

Rappaport, R. N. *et al*. (eds) (1982). *Families in Britain*. Routledge, London.

Robertson, J. (1984). Scenarios for lifestyle and health. *European Monographs in Health Education Research* **6**, 151–72.

Rubin, D. B. (1978). Multiple imputations in sample surveys—a phenomenological Bayesian approach to nonresponse. In *Imputation and editing of faulty or missing survey data* (eds F. Aziz and F. Scheuren). U.S. Dept. of Commerce, Bureau of the Census, Washington, D.C.

Rubin, D. B. (1979). *Handling non-response in sample surveys by multiple imputations*. Monograph prepared for U.S. Bureau of the Census.

RUHBC Working Papers (1985–6). No. 1 Telephone Survey Manual; No. 2 Report of a Study of the Edinburgh Women's Health Shop; No. 3 Sampling; No 4 West Lothian Food Survey; No. 5 ESRC study, development of an indicator of behavioural change. Papers by the research staff of the Research Unit in Health and Behavioural Change, Edinburgh, 1985–6.

Rutter, M. and Madje, J. (1976). *Cycles of disadvantage*. Heinemann, London.

Sykes, W. and Hoinville, G. (1985). *Telephone interviewing on a survey of social attitudes: a comparison with face-to-face procedures*. SCPR Survey Research Centre Publications, London.

Tanur, J. M. (1983). Methods for large-scale surveys and experiments. In *Sociological methodology* (ed. S. Leinhardt). Jossey-Bass Publishers, London.

Taylor, R. and Ford, G. (1981). Lifestyle and ageing: three traditions in lifestyle research. *Ageing and Society* **1**, 329–45.

Townsend, P. and Davidson, N. (1982). *Inequalities in health: the Black Report*. Penguin, Harmondsworth.

Tupek, A. R. and Richardson, W. J. (1978). Use of ratio estimates to compensate for non-response bias in certain economic surveys. In *Imputation and editing of faulty or missing survey data* (eds F. Aziz and F. Scheuren). U.S. Dept. of Commerce, Bureau of the Census, Washington, D.C.

Westman, M., Eden, D., and Shirom, A. (1985). Job stress, cigarette smoking and cessation: the conditioning effects of peer support. *Social Science and Medicine* **20**, 637–44.

WHO (1982). Lifestyles and their impact on health. Technical Discussion Paper, EUR/RC33/Tech.Disc./1. Copenhagen, WHO (EURO).

Wiley, J. A. and Comacho, T. C (1980). Life-style and future health: evidence from the Alameda County Study. *Preventive Medicine* **9**, 1–21.

Winship, C. and Mare, R. D. (1983). Structural equations and path analysis for discrete data. *American Journal of Sociology* **89**, 54–110.

22

A note on research priorities from participants in the Pitlochry Symposium on Health Behaviour

Research on health behaviour, applied to health promotion, should recognize the diverse 'realities' which are perceived by lay people, health professionals, and health researchers. This recognition should guide health researchers in their development of study areas, concepts, theories and methods in implementing research concerned with health promotion.

Researchers should recognize the 'contextual' nature of meaning. Behaviour related to health is itself found within the context of the general activities comprising the everyday life of people; this includes many settings: e.g. the home, the community, and the workplace. These social settings both constrain and enable opportunities for the development of concepts, meanings, and behaviour-related health. Furthermore, this context interacts with biological processes; it results in a complex interaction over a lifelong process.

A research environment should respond to and accept the diversity of existing research traditions which have led to a greater understanding of the public's health. Within the established research tradition, research in health promotion should emphasize:

1. The *application* of what we know to improve health.
2. The acceptance of appropriate and useful conceptual categories.
3. The appropriate application of these methods to issues of health promotion.

Research should pursue actively the development of *new* research initiatives which will lead to an improved understanding of how research may be applied towards the promotion of health. New research initiatives should emphasize:

1. The development of a theoretical and conceptual base; and a clarification of our conceptual categories.
2. Continuous, dynamic models and methods sensitive to social processes.
3. The linkage of theory and methods to health promotion.
4. A lifespan perspective, including emphases on the role of gender differences; the ageing process and behavioural change within the context of everyday life.

5. The need for different 'levels' of analysis/multiple units of analysis and the development of new methodologies.
6. The need for better 'indicators' of 'health'; individual indices and measures which have individual relevance.
7. The involvement of the 'community' in the research process.

As researchers we recognize that we are part of the process of implementing our research, that we are not passive 'observers' of health policy. Social policy itself is a 'contextual' factor in health promotion.

We should recognize that we have a role in public policy which impinges on the collective health, whether that policy enhances, maintains, or damages the public's health.

Research which adopts these guidelines assumes that:

1. Research on health promotion is not static and must deal with health as a process in which people's life context relates to the influence of social and economic factors on health. Research must monitor trends in society, economy, and technology in order to examine the nature of this dynamic process.
2. Research needed in the development of health promotion must be multi-disciplinary. Polarization, particularly between the medical and social sciences, must be avoided. There is a need for research on a broad canvas, which will provide a better understanding of factors that contribute to health.
3. Research should deal with the contribution of policy-makers. It needs to look at their expectations, both of the contribution they can make and perceived barriers to action and of the ideas they have about the expectations and priorities of the population. It is important to include an historical perspective on changes in policy over time.
4. Research is needed which is concerned with application, particularly with respect to generating public participation. Related to this is the need to examine the current health perceptions and practices of people, both lay and professional. This research should examine the ways in which people seek to maintain their own health, how this is influenced by social inequality and disadvantage, and by the availability of resources such as social support networks.

Arising from the Pitlochry meeting, several research questions should be noted, specifically with respect to gender, social networks, social policy, and social position.

Gender

1. What, if any, are the main gender differences in health attitudes, beliefs, and behaviours? Do they persist over time/across cultures?

2. How does the existing structure of health care organization influence gender-related health attitudes/beliefs/outcomes?
3. It might be interesting to look at exceptional situations, i.e. those who have aged successfully? e.g. women in male-dominated positions? men who are not successful in labour force, etc. There is a need to study male populations regarding health issues.

Social networks

1. There is a need to study social networks in terms of their role in social support, particularly with respect to the question of the 'quality' of the support.
2. What is the relationship between the instrumental and emotional components of social support?
3. The process and/or nature of social support need to be studied. What are the costs of receiving support and the costs of giving support?

Social policy

1. How is social policy a 'contextual' factor? That is, 'How does it affect researchers and how do researchers shape it?'
2. What kind of policy measures are needed to support changes in health behaviour in the population?
3. What kind of health promotion activities and research are needed to bring about changes in social policy?

Social position

1. We need to develop new classifications for social groups, involving concrete sets of characteristics relating to health—in relation to the labour market, family structures, and life-styles.
2. We need local neighbourhood studies which look at material and social conditions in which people live their everyday lives—the access to and command over resources related to health by local people, i.e. what are the opportunities for healthy behaviour and what are the resources necessary for healthy behaviour—how do these differ among/between classes, genders, ages, and communities.
3. Need to study the conditions under which individuals, classes, communities, and countries become energized to do something to promote their own and other people's, classes', communities' and countries' health.

Epilogue

Epilogue

M. STACEY

As I sit down to write the concluding chapter for the 'Pitlochry Symposium Book' I find myself in something of a quandary—several quandaries in fact. First, I have the notes I made for the final after-dinner speech on the work of the EACMR (European Advisory Committee on Medical Research) which I was originally asked to give. Then I have those notes modified to form an introduction to an overview of the symposium, which was how the platform (without warning) redefined my task on the first day, followed by somewhat staccato notes summing up the symposium, notes which become even more staccato as the Pitlochry revenge took hold. Second, I find that I have now a somewhat different (perhaps more mature) view of what went on at Pitlochry. Since then I have been to a meeting of the EACMR, addressed two other medical health-related meetings, and given a paper at the International Conference on Women's History in Amsterdam; and experienced the worst bout of 'flu I can remember for many a long day. Pitlochry appears as if through the wrong end of a telescope, but more sharply defined for all that. Third, it is not only I who have experienced changes: the EACMR is now the EACHR, that is to say it is now the European Advisory Committee on Health *Research, a change instituted by executive decision. The change had been in the air for a good while, but was always blocked (so far as I know mostly by medical men) when discussed on the committee or any of its subcommittees. Not only that, the terms of reference of the committee have been restated. Finally, I do not know which of the papers that I heard given are to be included as chapters in the book and how they may be revised.*

In these circumstances how should I proceed? The most tempting solution was to write and say that I cannot now write this conclusion unless you give me more time and send me the revisions and then I will write a paper which sums them up critically and, hopefully, constructively. A second possibility would be to write a conclusion which takes account of institutional changes in footnotes but concealed all the personal and public histories of the past two months and appeared perfectly rational and systematic and apparently followed appropriate scientific canons. My fingers on the typewriter felt heavy as I contemplated how such an account would go. I decided it was not 'me' and rationalized that quickly by deciding option two was scientistic and not scientific. Furthermore I soon convinced myself that this was a reason and not a rationalization. The third option was born out of the practical and intellectual difficulties of the first two. It is the option I am following, namely to comment on the symposium as I now see it in retrospect, to relate that to the work of the EACHR as that is now constituted and to see what the editors think of the result.

This revision of what a concluding overview ought conventionally to be bears some cousinship to what I had proposed to do with the after-dinner speech, had the Pitlochry revenge not struck. Giving that speech had already given me problems in anticipation. So far as the first assignment was concerned I had asked myself who would want to hear about the EACMR after three intense days incarcerated discussing health behaviour? The tradition of the after-dinner speech and the EACMR did not seem to go well together and it also did not seem to be like 'me'. Men, I said to myself, make after-dinner speeches, the successful ones inducing laughter over the port. I've never worried about doing jobs conventionally assigned to men except when they mean that I am expected to behave like a man in the sense of denying my womanhood. The laughter in after-dinner speeches is most commonly called forth by risquee, dirty, and often downright sexist jokes. The after-dinner speech is a male tradition out of the male culture, part of the supporting apparatus of male domination; the women listen while the men speak, reaffirming the excellence of the men and the groups they belong to. But I am a woman and I try to fight like a woman (Stacey 1982) and to make speeches as a woman, so dirty jokes are out. I long since refused to be recruited as an honorary male, although the temptations continue and the alternative path is uncomfortable. The problem of how to make the work of the EACMR entertaining was then replaced by the more severe problem of talking after dinner about the symposium to people who had already heard three concluding addresses that afternoon and really just wanted to relax.

There was of course an alternative model for after-dinner speeches, the Mansion House model, where the great political leader dicourses on party and nation. Was I supposed to do that sort of thing? A rousing call 'forward to better European research on health promotion with the EACMR!'? If so, on several counts that was impossible. This drew to mind the other thing about after-dinner speeches: namely their ritualistic and ceremonial nature which, like everything else about them has the effect of reaffirming the elite and the hierarchy. The speech is made, there is polite clapping, the brandy and cigars are turned to with relief.

I had therefore decided for all these reasons that I would not make a conventional speech, or conventional remarks, but, taking a leaf from the women's movement, would share with the participants my understanding of what the symposium had been about, and explain what I had to do on the EACMR, and the work the WHO EURO staff had to do, and to ask for the diners' view and advice on these matters—turning the whole thing into a relaxed discussion if participants had been willing to respond.

It is in that spirit that I shall write this conclusion. My only regret is that I shall not get the instant feedback that I had initially hoped for, but if the paper is *published it will hopefully flow in gradually through the usual informal and formal academic channels.*

Looking back now to how I see the symposium, what was its value, what are the problems we have to face, both intellectual and practical? First of all the disparate schools of thought and traditions of research which were represented was quite striking. How members found it difficult to talk to and comprehend each other, was the second impression, closely linked with the first. The differences were partly of discipline, partly of method, partly of politics or ideology. Among the medically qualified there were divisions between clinicians and epidemiologists; among the latter there were those who accepted the broad outlines of the discipline as received and at least one who had ceased to accept them. Among the social scientists there were those who worked with quantitative methods and others with qualitative; one got somewhat the impression that those who worked qualitatively also worked quantitatively, or at least appreciated the place and importance (if also the limitations) of the quantitative method, but that the same was not true, or not to the same extent, of those who worked quantitatively; for them scientific method was important and in research, such as that associated with health behaviour, scientific method meant numerate methods. If those who were involved in practice, whether as clinicians, as community physicians, or health care planners, were impatient of researchers who were not practitioners, they did not show it.

The methodological differences reflected, but were by no means isomorphic with, the focus of research, as to whether the focus should be upon the individual or the collectivity; and where the focus should be upon the collectivity; what form it should take. Epidemiologists and community physicians see themselves as quite distinct from clinicians in so far as the former deal with the health and illness of populations, while the latter are inevitably in a one-to-one relation with their patients. Sociologists, on the other hand, taking the collectivity as their subject of study, are more inclined to stress the importance of shared meanings and behaviours and to look beyond the individual for causes of illness and modes of health promotion. While a more individualistic focus can be expected to arise from branches of biomedicine with its origins in individual treatment, underlying differences of ideology also emerged. Once again these divisions to some extent cross-cut each other; that is to say, as with the issue of method and individual or collective focus, so with the ideological differences. Those whose work concentrated on individual behaviour or belief and its relationship to health and illness outcomes were more inclined to make underlying assumptions about the autonomy of the individual and her/his ability to control her/his own life. Those who approached the question more from a collective point of view were more inclined to observe and to stress in their explanations the constraints upon individuals as to the extent to which they might adopt healthy behaviour and the extent to which circumstances quite outside their control, *from workplace hazards to war, might affect their chances of a healthy life. At the level of values also, there were differences as to the morality of risk-taking behaviour, some risks being inevitable in life and the consequences of constant risk-avoidance being unknown, just as differences in the level of risk-taking among people in various life-cycle stages were not fully understood. The policy implications of the different approaches are considerable: the underlying question was not really addressed, although often touched upon. If the stress in health promotion is to be upon individual actions and behaviour then one set of policies follow; if the stress is to be upon the constraints which prevent healthy behaviour, then policies have to be primarily addressed to societal arrangements of one sort or another. In practice, neither in research nor policy-making are the issues quite as stark as that, but the question of alternative emphases is clear.*

Among divisions of the kind already discussed there were many cross-cutting threads. Furthermore, the differences were inter-national or cross-national; there was no sense in which the nationals of one country all lined up behind a particular approach, although there were distinctive and valuable contributions which came from different countries. The sense one had of the seminar was that, above all these differences, was a shared wish to come to terms with the problems and issues associated with health behaviour and health promotion. Had this not been the case there would not have been such lively discussion continuing until the end of the sessions.

For my part, what was most valuable about the seminar was just this confrontation among the various schools of thought. It seemed to me that in the course of the seminar the notion of health behaviour was extended in a variety of ways beyond a narrowly conceived individualistic approach. It was extended to include the idea that health behaviour was related to the ideas and concepts that people have about health, illness, and their causations; that these vary systematically by gender and by social class and status. The notion of health behaviours also was extended to include the opportunities and constraints which individuals and groups experience who live in particular geographic locations in particular historic periods. One mode of researching such ideas was to bring the various methodologies together to examine the health, health behaviour, and concepts of the residents of distinct localities. But these would also need to take account of the experiences of residents in times past, such as from war, occupation, pogrom, or discrimination.

The implications of this extension included the notion that for health promotion one needs research which will offer an understanding not only of how people behave with regard to health but why they behave in that way; not only in terms of what their health beliefs are, but why they might have those beliefs; and, most importantly, how these beliefs are rooted in their individual and collective experiences. Without these understandings health promotion programmes are likely to lack salience for those to whom they are directed, and thus either create unproductive (indeed possibly destructive) anxiety among the recipients or merely be totally ignored as irrelevant.

Associated with this was the implication that research for health promotion requires interdisciplinary co-operation, which implies that researchers of different disciplines should understand, learn to respect and to work with each others' models. This has to be a mutual learning; no one discipline, or group of disciplines, can be expected to act as handmaidens of others. There has been some tendency in the past for the biomedical to claim paramountcy. The empirical evidence before the Pitlochry group made it plain that when it comes to health promotion, the knowledge and understanding, the research models and the conceptual approach of the social sciences is as critical as that of the biomedical sciences, including epidemiology; that none can do the task without the others.

At this juncture I should turn to the way in which the symposium relates to the work of WHO EURO and specifically to the EACHR and the work I have to do there. As a number of participants said to me during the symposium, what is EACMR, as it then was? What, they might also have said (had it been mentioned on the programme), is ERAP? At the outset of 1985, when I was invited to sit on EACMR by the Regional Director, I had no idea either. Whereas, when I was invited to serve on the General Medical Council I had some idea of what it was about in terms of regulating the medical profession, although it was a pretty shadowy body in my mind which I envisaged as composed of grey-haired old men, the EACMR I had never heard of. The World Health Organization I knew a bit about and also that it was divided into regions and that there was a European Region, but there my knowledge ended. From the fog which the grey paper created, referred to by a participant during the seminar, sometimes real people like Ilona Kickbusch emerged bringing with them a shaft of intelligible light. As it so happened I had never had a conversation with Raymond Illsley about the Committee although he had served on it for some four years before me.

The European Advisory Committee on Medical Research (EACMR) was established in 1976. The report which defined its tasks at that time was headed 'The Role of the Regional Office for Europe in the Development and Co-ordination of Biomedical Research'. The committee was:

1. *To assist in the co-ordination of national research programmes in order to improve the efficiency and effectiveness of health services in Europe.*
2. *To identify problem areas and establish priorities, particularly with regard to health services research.*
3. *To develop research components of long-term programmes in the Regional Office.*
4. *To develop and maintain contacts with existing research co-ordinating bodies in Europe and the appropriate units at WHO headquarters.*

In 1983 the specification changed:

1. *To assess the soundness of the scientific basis of the WHO programme in Europe, its capacity for innovation and its contribution to the improvement of health.*
2. *To advise the Regional Director of research priorities.*
3. *To serve as an intermediary between health administrators and the scientific community.*

In February 1986 the terms of reference were reviewed. (It transpired that none had ever been formally adopted as such.) The terms were grouped under three headings:

1. *Advising the Regional Director on the scientific basis for the regional policy for health for all, and especially on the research to support this policy in member countries and the Region as a whole.*
2. *Helping the Regional Office make such research for health known to and accepted by the research community and governments in member states, as well as by inter-governmental and non-governmental organizations active in this field in Europe.*
3. *Advising the Regional Director on the scientific basis and research components of all programmes under the responsibility of the Regional Office, along with the quality of their implementation (Document 1097d).*

These changes since 1976 can be seen to reflect the unquestioned primacy of biomedicine and the curative approach at the outset and the move toward not only prevention but the promotion of positive health which has followed from Director General Mahler's speech of 1976, the acceptance by the World Health Assembly in 1977 of the target of health for all by the year 2000 (HFA 2000 for short), and the declaration of Alma-Ata in 1978 stressing the importance of primary health care.

In accordance with this policy the European Region adopted Targets for Health For All in 1984 (WHO 1985). Five targets, 13–17, are concerned with life styles conducive to health and are those to which deliberations of this seminar might be expected to contribute. Target 32 is related to research strategies which will contribute to the goal of health for all. This is the target which is of particular concern to the EACHR which, as we have seen, has been modified and is being redirected one might say towards notions of health promotion rather than cure or even disease prevention.

The committee members are appointed to achieve a geographic and professional balance and a balance between different kinds of research (basic, clinical, health care systems, and behavioural and social sciences) and designed to be able to cover research policy, administration, and funding. There are 16 members, each from a different country, drawn from the 33 member nations. Each adviser serves for four years, although some may be reappointed after a break. At any one meeting there are probably as many officers in attendance from WHO EURO and WHO HQ as there are advisers. The advisers include academic researchers and health care administrators; their closeness to political and policy involvements therefore varies. There are currently four social scientists of whom three are sociologists (of varying kinds) and one a health economist. This is a larger number than formerly and reflects the changes of emphasis which I mentioned earlier.

The committee meets annually for one week usually in Copenhagen, with sub-committees in between for those who have the misfortune to be picked. The members are temporary advisers to the Regional Director who are appointed by him and sit with the consent of their governments. The real work is of course done by the staff—not that the work the advisers do during and between meetings is not pretty arduous for as long as it lasts.

Perhaps the best way to convey this is to describe a meeting. One finds oneself sitting at one of two sides of a long table in a conference room with the top table having the chairperson, vice chair, Regional Director, Committee Secretary and other senior officials. Facing the top table are the glass fronted cabins of the translators. This is not one of those international meetings, I am happy to say, where one has to sit behind one's national flag, for we are not here as nationals but as advisers to the Regional Director. The international character of the meeting and the need for translation means that there have to be particular techniques for speaking, the process of catching the chairperson's eye is augmented by having to wait for the light to signal that the translators are ready. All this tends to make exchanges somewhat ponderous. Increasingly many delegates speak in English which is good for me, but leaves the English translators with less to do. The standard of translation is excellent and rapid. Sitting at the table I once again find I'm among predominantly male company, among biomedics, some clinicians, some administrators, some community physicians or epidemiologists, but most biomedically based.

The major input from members will be reports of the reviews that they have made of areas of work of the Office as to its academic soundness and sufficiency as regards its research base. Generally two members report on each area and perhaps two major areas are investigated and discussed each year. There will also be reports from and discussions about other European bodies responsible for or undertaking research. WHO has itself very little money directly to fund research; most work therefore is in the area of encouraging bodies to support work which falls within the WHO EURO research priorities.

The major work of the committee over recent years has been to develop the European Research Action Plan (ERAP) in support of the Health for All targets which I mentioned earlier. This flows from target 32 about developing appropriate research to help achieve the HFA goals. This plan has now been worked out in its first draft; it indicates areas where there is a lack of research data; what barriers there are to achieving research for the various targets and what sort of research may be needed to develop an adequate research base. As a draft it will *be presented to the Regional Advisory Committee and, after amendment, to the Regional Council; it will then be sent to member states, research bodies, both national and international, for their comments. This process will start in the summer of 1986. The final plan will be agreed in September of 1987.* *

What does all this mean and what is its relevance to this seminar? First of all, of course, the seminar is closely associated with the work of Ilona Kickbusch's sector of work within the European Office. Its deliberations will constitute part of the research base which informs her work. As part of the whole of the activities with which she and her colleagues are involved, it will at some point be the subject of a review by the EACHR. At this point other members of that committee, not involved in this area of research, will get to know what work is going on there. In that context I would be prepared to guess that the differences which have loomed among us this week, sometimes appearing quite large and sometimes distressing researchers whose life work or current major commitments seemed to be coming under severe criticism, these differences would become as nothing compared to the joint effort that would have to be made to ensure that work associated with health information, health behaviour, concepts and promotion should be taken seriously and properly understood.

Secondly, European members of this seminar will have an interest in watching out for the ERAP* and commenting on it. Whatever we may think as individuals about the 'realpolitik' of HFA2000, there is no doubt at all that in this, as in other areas, Mahler's initiative can have a liberating effect. Just as some member states have been able to get health budgets upgraded because of WHO leadership, so there is a chance for those who wish to see a health rather than an illness orientation to get the balance of research expenditure changed in favour of, inter alia, the kind of work that researchers here present are interested in, competent at, and which has hitherto been seriously underfunded in relation to more strictly biomedical research. However, there is no fairy godmother in the shape of WHO or anyone else who will wave a wand and make these resources available. It will be up to us, as members of the research community, to insist that our governments pay attention to the document which will be open for consultation; to make sure it is made widely known to funding bodies so that it may influence their deliberations; and to press for more appropriate machinery to be established where this is necessary. For my part, at this stage, I shall find one of the contradictions of membership of EACHR coming upon me, namely that while one is not a national representative and therefore does not in any way act as a representative of government on EACHR, nevertheless WHO expects members to help to forward EACHR policies within their own countries and among their own research communities. In much the same way it was, I suppose, that I was asked to come to this conference: partly because I have spent*

* By the time the research plan was finally agreed, its name had been changed to Research for Health for All. (R.H.F.A.)

about 25 years working on various sorts of health research and might therefore be expected to have a research contribution to make; and partly because of the inevitable political (small p) consequences of serving on the EACHR. For my own part I would not do that rather hard work, cynical as I am as most are about international collaboration in this world of ours at this time, if I did not think we had to go on pegging away wherever a channel for some hope and improvement presents itself. Certainly the work of this seminar helped me in the work which I was called on to do at Copenhagen.

References

Stacey, M. (1982). Social sciences and the State: fighting like a woman. British Sociological Association Presidential Address. *Sociology* **16**, 406–21.

World Health Organization (1985). *Targets for health for all: Targets in support of the European regional strategy for health for all*. WHO Regional Office for Europe, Copenhagen.

Index

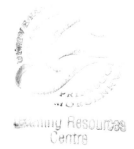